Positive Paths to Wellbeing

Your journey to a
calmer, happier, healthier life

Marie Paterson

Published in 2024 by Balcomie Books
Copyright © 2024 Marie Paterson

ISBN Paperback: 978-1-7384526-2-0
ISBN Ebook: 978-1-7384526-1-3

Important Note:
This book is not intended as a substitute for health
advice or treatment. Any person with a condition requiring
medical attention should consult a qualified medical
practitioner.

Illustrations: Emily Carr

A CIP catalogue record of this book is available
from the British Library.

Dedication

To everyone I have ever learnt from, thank you for your
part in my journey. I could not have done it without you.

Contents

Introduction

What is wellbeing? We hear the term used many times a day on the news, the radio and in social media. Since the pandemic, wellbeing has become a focal point of many policies and initiatives, as being isolated during lockdown was detrimental to most people's wellbeing. But what does it mean?

The *Oxford English Dictionary* defines it as follows: 'With reference to a person or community: the state of being healthy, happy or prosperous; physical, psychological or moral welfare.'

I was not really sure I understood that explanation, so I wondered what ChatGPT, the artificial intelligence system, would say. First it gave me a long description, which was rather helpful but not what I wanted, so I asked it for a shorter definition, and this was the response:

'Wellbeing is a state of overall health, happiness and contentment that encompasses physical, mental, emotional and social aspects of life.'

I much prefer that answer, as it's so much easier to understand. That ChatGPT is good! Maybe I should give up writing this book right now! Well, you can see that I did keep going, and I am delighted that you are holding my book in your hands. If your definition of wellbeing is different from the one above, congratulations – we are all unique individuals, and this book celebrates that fact. It will help you look at your life, not someone else's, and help you find your optimal wellbeing in a way that works for you. So read on and find your own unique positive paths to wellbeing.

My journey to becoming a wellbeing trainer and coach started 20 years ago, when my boss at the time gave me a book called *The 7 Habits of Highly Effective People* by Stephen R Covey. I was a bit concerned that she felt I needed to read this book, but I came to discover she just loved sharing the wisdom that was contained in the pages, and it wasn't a reflection of how she felt about my work. Phew! And I can honestly say that it changed my life in many ways, ultimately leading to me writing this book.

The first change that *7 Habits* brought about was to how I thought and behaved as a parent. At the time I read the book, I was mum to 13- and 11-year-old daughters. And as my elder daughter was entering the teenage years, I naturally found that I was having some arguments with her. I had always considered myself to be a patient person. I had been a teacher of secondary school pupils (aged 11–18) and I didn't lose my temper with them even when they were behaving badly. But I found I was starting to lose self-control with my teenager. She would be annoyed with me, I would get annoyed with her and raise my voice and she would raise hers right back, and that would escalate with me losing the plot and afterwards I would feel utterly ashamed of my behaviour. But did I blame myself? I don't think I did. I blamed her! After all, I had always been a patient person until then, so it must be her fault. You get my logic. But when I read *The 7 Habits of Highly Effective People*, a key principle struck me. Now this was nothing complex, just plain old common sense really, but sadly it had been missing from my interactions with my daughter at the time. The principle is one that Covey attributes to Victor Frankl, author of *Man's Search for Meaning*.[1] Frankl was an Austrian psychiatrist and Auschwitz survivor. The principle is 'between stimulus and response there is a space, and in that space is our power to choose'. This is not a complicated statement but just a reminder that when something happens we do have the power to choose what to do next, although we often forget that. We are not pre-programmed robots, but sometimes we act that way. The stimulus was my daughter raising her voice to me, as she pushed back against some constraint I was imposing on her 13-year-old lifestyle. The response was me telling her to jolly well do as she was told and stop arguing with me, followed by annoyance from her as she struggled to exert her natural desire for more independence. And then I would get more annoyed and so on in a downward spiral of anger, stress, sadness and frustration, and then she would stomp off with a passing 'Mother!' For me, as my anger subsided, I would feel a deep, deep shame that I had lost my temper and modelled a terrible way to respond to a disagreement between us. How could I expect her to turn into a calm, rational, thoughtful adult if that was the role model her mother presented?

And then to the rescue came Stephen R Covey. I got to meet him once, which was a great pleasure. I had heard that he was speaking at an event in London so I got in touch with the organiser and explained that I was a massive fan and could I come along and just sneak in at the back. And amazingly she said yes. How kind was that? It just goes to show that if you don't ask, you don't get. When I arrived, all excited about getting to sneak into the back of this large auditorium, I found that they had put me on a table at the front, so while Covey was giving his talk I was about a metre away from him. In the interval I managed to get a quick word. I was rather star struck!

Anyway, I digress. How did Covey rescue me? When I read his explanation about the space between stimulus and response, I realised that I was not using it. I was going down an automatic response pathway: raised voice from daughter, instant shout from me. I was not pausing and thinking about what the right response would be. What would be the response if I wanted her to learn how to communicate her frustration effectively, if I wanted her to develop self-control (which clearly her mother had lost the plot with)?

So what did I do? At the end of the chapter I had been reading, I vowed that I would start to think more when the stimulus happened. That I would take a micro pause and choose a better response. That I would choose my words, tone of voice and body language rather than go down the auto-pilot route, and what do you know? When she got annoyed with me and I didn't respond in my old ways but instead stayed calm, she calmed down too. I can honestly say from that day on we never got into another similar down-ward spiral. Sure we disagreed about some things but we talked them through much more calmly. As you can imagine, the fact that this nugget of information in *The 7 Habits* led to a major improvement with my teenage daughter made me fall in love with the book and also the whole field of self-development.

I then got rather obsessed with learning more about self-development and I was lucky enough to train to deliver a workshop on the 7 Habits (under licence), which I ran a few times a year for 10 years to over 600 delegates in total.

It wasn't only self-development that I got hooked on; I also got very interested in physical health too. As I worked in community services in the NHS, I was involved with various projects, and many of them had something in common, namely trying to support people with long-term health issues. Whether that was heart disease, diabetes, lung problems or the more general term of frailty, one thing was certain to me – I didn't want to end up with any of these conditions. Now obviously I could not change my genetic predisposition to various illnesses, but I could have an influence on many of the contributing factors, such as what I ate, how active I was, and how I managed stress. I got very interested in looking at the factors that could help me live a healthy life for as long as possible. I started studying for a nutrition certificate, became an exercise trainer for older adults and took courses in counselling, coaching, mindfulness, and Acceptance and Commitment Therapy.

Now you may have come across some people in the media who are obsessed with living very long lives by experimenting with various new treatments, supplements and medications. That is not for me. I just want to find the balance between enjoying life and maximising my health, and most importantly, keeping physically and mentally fit for as long as possible. Maybe I will be an amazing 100-year-old, or maybe I won't make 70. Who knows? But I want to be able to walk up hills, run for a bus, lift my suitcase into the overhead locker on a plane all by myself, fit into the same clothes, and enjoy my work, my family and friends for as long as possible. To put it bluntly, I want to have a long, healthy life and a quick death. Of course, I have no control over so many things that will influence my lifespan, but I do have control over some of the things that affect my healthspan (my healthy years of life).

When I left my job in the NHS to start up my own coaching and training business, I was passionate about helping others – helping them to live calmer, happier, healthier lives. So my business focused on sharing the knowledge I had gained over the years. I decided to bring all of my learning into a framework called *Positive Paths to Wellbeing*. I then developed the framework into a two-day workshop which I translated into an online course during the pandemic. I have since incorporated *Positive Paths to Wellbeing* into a team wellbeing programme and I support team members to improve their individual wellbeing as well as develop a culture of wellbeing in their organisation.

I am not sure when I decided to turn the course into this book, but the progression from workshop to online course to book seemed fairly logical. Writing it has been a steep learning curve and I am delighted that it is at last in the hands of my readers. Thank you so much for taking the time to read the book. I hope your time will be well rewarded.

Positive Paths to Wellbeing consists of eight paths which are broken down into 22 milestones, and you can see the names of each one in the infographic at the end of this introduction. Each milestone provides you with information on how to look after your wellbeing but, more importantly, it also asks you to reflect on your own personal situation. We are all different. We are unique individuals. No two people have exactly the same genetics or upbringing. Even identical twins with identical genetics will have variations in the turning on and off of their genes (epigenetics), plus some variation in their upbringing. So make sure you focus on you as an individual as you read through the book. There are places to stop and reflect as you go through the paths. You might like to get a fresh notebook and have that with you as you read. Only by stopping and answering the questions will you really benefit from the exploration of the paths. Otherwise, it is a bit like buying a travel guidebook to Peru, reading it from cover to cover, but then never actually setting foot in the country. And unless you answer the questions honestly, you won't gain maximum benefit from them. But before you go any further, a word of warning: if you feel that thinking deeply about your physical and mental wellbeing could be traumatic for you, then this might not be the time to read this book. Maybe you can find a counsellor or therapist to work with on the issues that are concerning you. That may not be easy to access due to the cost, so maybe there is someone you trust who you can confide in, such as a family member, friend or your GP. There are also many organisations that can help with the issues that life throws at us with lots of people willing and wanting to help; so please do seek these out if you need help. Don't suffer alone; there are people out there to support you.

However, if you are not in a traumatic situation and want to learn from the wisdom of others, get ready to dive in. Over the years I learnt how to manage my behaviour better by learning from the leaders, authors and experts that I have followed, and I now share those thoughts and ideas with you in this book. No one is perfect, certainly not me, and life is very much a work in progress, but to me it makes sense to use the wisdom of others to make life that bit easier. I hope that this book provides you with some food for thought to help you in your journey through life. I am not a researcher, a doctor or a wellbeing guru, but what I am is an educator. Educators help others to learn and that is what my book is here to do, to help you learn more about your wellbeing. So now if you are ready to make a difference to your life, grab a notebook and pen and let's get going – happy exploring!

Infographic

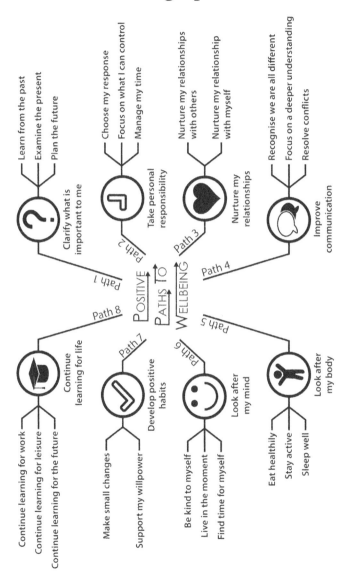

POSITIVE PATHS TO WELLBEING

Path 1
- Learn from the past
- Examine the present
- Plan the future
- Clarify what is important to me

Path 2 — Take personal responsibility
- Choose my response
- Focus on what I can control
- Manage my time

Path 3 — Nurture my relationships
- Nurture my relationships with others
- Nurture my relationship with myself

Path 4 — Improve communication
- Recognise we are all different
- Focus on a deeper understanding
- Resolve conflicts

Path 5 — Look after my body
- Eat healthily
- Stay active
- Sleep well

Path 6 — Look after my mind
- Be kind to myself
- Live in the moment
- Find time for myself

Path 7 — Develop positive habits
- Make small changes
- Support my willpower

Path 8 — Continue learning for life
- Continue learning for work
- Continue learning for leisure
- Continue learning for the future

Path 1
Clarify what is important to me

'The best way to predict your future is to create it.'
Abraham Lincoln

1:A – Learn from the past

Today is the start of a journey of self-discovery. In this book you will learn many principles and tools that will help you live a calmer, happier, healthier life. I really hope it will be an uplifting journey of self-discovery, learning and action. I know that as you work through the book and reflect on your life, you will discover how to get more of the things you love into your days. No one wants to get towards the end of their life and have a dawning realisation that they have not prioritised the people and activities that really matter. But it is never too late, whatever your age, to get some clarity on those important things and to start planning for change. Certainly for me that is a continuing process. Taking a pause at different times of the year and different stages of life to just check in with myself and to ask what, right now, is important to me. So enough of the preamble; let's get going!

The first of our eight paths is *Clarify what is important to me*, and to start this we are going to have a quick look into the past. In this first exercise I am asking you to think about the positive things that have happened in your life so far. Sometimes as life marches on we don't reflect on what has been important to us, and over time many things get forgotten. So I want you to divide your life into at least three sections, maybe more. Have a think about the natural transition times. For me the key transitions are primary school, secondary school, university, children at home, then after children left. Decide what are the key sections in your life and jot them down in your notebook.

Now I want you to spend some time thinking about all the positive things that happened in each of these sections of your life. Please do not dwell on anything negative. There are some questions below to prompt you, but don't let these questions limit your imagination; they are just there to help if you are struggling to think back. Try to write down lots of different reflections and reminiscences.

For each key section of my life:
- What was I good at?
- Who were the people I enjoyed being with?
- What were the landmark days?
- What made me happy?
- What skills did I develop?
- What made me proud?
- Who did I help?
- What groups was I part of?
- What made me laugh?

How did you find that? Did you remember some things you had not thought about for ages? For me I remembered the days when I did Irish dancing; I gave up at 13 or you might have seen me on Riverdance! I reminisced about when my children were young, and I thought about all the new things I have learnt since I started my own business. It highlighted that the key areas of my life are my family and friends, my health, my hobbies and continued learning. When I reflect on that list it certainly feels right and is helpful for prioritising my focus and time. There are so many things we can do and because we can't do them all we need to make time for the things that are truly important. Knowing what is important to you can help you plan for the days, months and even years ahead.

So what did you learn about what is important to you? I want you to spend a few more minutes answering that important question. Are there any things from the past that you would like to get back into your life now? Any changes that you would like to make? Or maybe it has made you realise that there are things that take up a lot of your time that you could stop doing. Obviously we all need to prioritise our work so that we have enough money to cover our most basic needs such as a home to live in and food to eat, but it can be easy to fill up our lives with activities that we don't really enjoy and that don't fulfil us. In this time of the internet when it is easy to spend so much time on our screens, perhaps there is something that would be better for us – more enjoyable or more fulfilling – that we would like to find time for. Realistically what can you stop or do less of so that you can start that activity?

I know for me I spend too much time on my phone, but by removing some of the apps, I have cut down on screen time and mostly use it now for work and practical life admin – the banking app is very handy! I know I could reduce it further, but I want to emphasise here that *Positive Paths to Wellbeing* is not about being 'perfect', whatever that may mean to you. It is not about having the perfect home, job, family, hair, whatever else springs to mind. *Positive Paths to Wellbeing* is about being more mindful about what would help you to be calmer, happier and healthier and then prioritising to get more of those activities into your life. So don't beat yourself up for spending too long on your phone, having an untidy house or not eating only organic whole food. Let's ditch the aim for perfection but be more conscious about what lifts us up and makes us feel good. We will get back to this topic again in Path 6 but for now just make a note of anything that seems to be important to you, but that you don't do enough of.

1:B – Examine the present

In milestone 1:A we focused on learning from the past and now we will think about how life is at the moment. You will see on page 15 the Wheel of Wellbeing with 12 areas of life that impact on how we feel, both mentally and physically. I want you to think about each segment, then score how **satisfied** you are with that area of your life right now. It is very personal to you and does not reflect your achievements in that area, only your current level of satisfaction. For example, if you are not in work or a career for whatever reason, such as because you are a parent, studying or retired, and you are completely satisfied with that, it gets a score of 10. If you don't have any hobbies, because work and family take up your time and you are quite satisfied with that, again it would get a high score. Don't compare yourself to anyone else, just think about how satisfied you are right now in each of the 12 areas. Where there are areas you would like to change, they will get a lower score.

Now take a few minutes to reflect on each segment and give it that score out of 10. Feel free to make some notes too as you go around the wheel. This exercise can give you some deep insights into your life if you take the time to think carefully. Remember you haven't been to Peru if you only read the guidebook – you need to go there to experience it, and the same is true of this exercise. Reading the titles of the 12 segments is like reading the guidebook. Spending time thinking deeply about how satisfied you are in each area and making some notes is like visiting Peru! So don't skip over this exercise. It will help you to identify if there are any changes you would like to make to improve your wellbeing.

Note – Most areas of the Wheel of Wellbeing are self-explanatory.

For finances don't forget to include planning for the future and retirement. For community have a think about your neighbours, the area you live in, any groups that you are a member of, any religious community you are part of, any charities that you support.

Wheel of Wellbeing

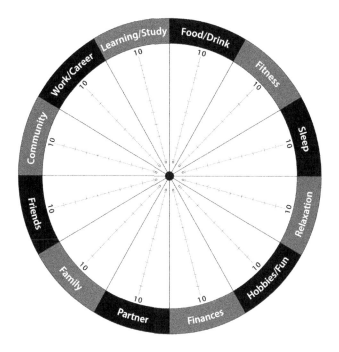

Once you have completed the wheel, spend some time thinking about what ideas you can put into action to increase your satisfaction score in each segment. Take the time to note them down. The Wheel of Wellbeing is going to be an important tool in helping you make changes in the future, so do take your time over it. I don't expect you to immediately launch into making changes in your life. But it might be interesting to underline one thing, just one thing, that would make the biggest difference to your life if you worked on that idea. Think about how you can start to put that idea into action. As we work through the rest of the paths, they will help you to identify some helpful actions, so don't feel you have to make any changes yet. Remember we are still at the start of the journey.

Now at this point I want to caution against trying to make lots of changes all at once as you will only get overwhelmed. It is better to make small plans that you stick to, than to set ambitious goals that overwhelm you and are unsustainable.

When I completed the Wheel of Wellbeing a few years ago, one of the areas I wanted to improve was my physical health. I decided to start a regime of exercises in the morning and of course I started with great enthusiasm. I developed a regime of six or seven different exercises and they took me about seven or eight minutes. But then in my typically over-enthusiastic way I started to add in more exercises. (Hey, look at me; I've got this!) And then it started to take about 15–20 minutes and guess what? I stopped doing them. Completely. Not even the seven-minute version. Twenty minutes was just too much for me in the morning. It interfered with my morning routine far too much and I didn't enjoy it. And my good habit petered out.

However, knowing that this was really very important for my ageing body, I decided to start back at the seven to eight minutes again, varying the exercises over a few mornings, and I have managed to stick to that for about five mornings a week for a number of years. As a result, I feel stronger than ever and I rarely get a sore back, which I used to get quite regularly. I even have noticeable biceps for the first time in my life!

So my top tips are don't over-commit, be realistic and find changes that you can fit into your everyday life. Oh, and don't start planning too much just yet – we still have lots more to discover. But don't let me stop you either if you are itching to make a small change.

Finally, before we move on to the next milestone, take a minute to appreciate all you have achieved in your life so far. The education you worked hard for. The work you have done. The people you have made a difference to and the skills you have developed. You have achieved so much already and there are many more opportunities ahead on your journey through life. Having clarity about what is important to you will help you to embrace them.

1:C – Plan the future

If you have completed the exercises so far you will have looked at the past and had a trip down memory lane. You will have analysed the present and maybe started to think about something you might like to change. We are now going to take a peek into the future.

I want you to imagine that you have won £5 million on the lottery. I don't know if that sounds wonderful or fills you with horror, but please bear with me. Take some time to think about what you would do with the money. Try to write down at least five ideas. It can be anything, so use your imagination. It can be things for yourself or others. Maybe you would give some away, buy a big house, give up work, start a business, get a fancy car or whatever you think would be right for you.

Now think about each of those ideas and ask yourself why you would choose to spend the money that way. Keep digging down and asking why, over and over again, until you feel you have really got to the heart of it.

Let me give you an example. An attendee at one of my workshops said she would spend some of the money on a big family holiday. When she asked herself why, she said she wanted to spend more time with her young family. She asked herself 'why' again and came up with the answer that what she really wanted was to have a relaxed time, playing with her children. And on further digging down she realised she just wanted to have more fun with her kids and that was really the heart of the matter. One of her children had said to her recently, 'Mummy, you only laugh when we are on holiday.' That really touched her heart (and mine too). Then the question she needed to ask herself was could she do that crucially important thing – in her case having fun with her kids – without £5 million. Of course she could. She resolved there and then to go home that evening and have some fun.

I know it is tempting to skip over these exercises – I have done that myself – but do take the time to dig down deep and discover some of the things that are truly important to you. Get to the heart of it. Then ask yourself if you can do those things without lots of money. I have done this exercise with so many people and they almost always say YES. I think you will find that you can too. Now of course you would not be able to buy that big house or go on a world cruise without the money, but if the real reason you wanted these things was to spend more time with your family, you can easily have their company without £5 million.

These three exercises – the happy memories from the past, the Wheel of Wellbeing and the lottery win – have hopefully revealed to you some of the things that are deeply important to you. You can now use any insights they have revealed in the next exercise. Read through the information below and answer the questions with as much detail as feels right for you. I want you to use your imagination to picture a day six months from now. Your life is feeling good. The sun is shining and you are relaxed and happy. Try and picture yourself in control, confident and calm.

- What is that date?
- Where are you?
- What are you doing?
- Who are you with?
- What is different about you compared to today?

Now if you want to write anything down, please do. But don't worry if you don't. We are not going to finalise this exercise, this 'vision of the future', until the end of the book. But I do want you to know that we will be working towards it, and I want you to jot down any ideas you have about this vision as we go through the remaining seven paths. In coaching I help people to think ahead, to have a vision of what they would like to be different in their life. Often it is something connected to work, like getting a promotion, changing jobs, starting a business or retiring. Sometimes it is related to improving relationships or it might be a personal challenge like completing a qualification. Other times it might be health related like getting fitter or eating more healthily. Everyone has different starting points and different goals and aspirations. The important thing is to be aware of what those goals are and to start taking action to get there. I also recommend that you don't only focus on the destination but aim to enjoy the journey along the way. Being curious about what you are learning, what you are changing and how that is impacting on your life can make the journey as important, if not more so, than the destination.

Do remember we are just at the very start of the journey through the book so you don't need to make any great plans at the moment. You are just beginning to think about the factors that affect your wellbeing and if there is anything you would like to change. In Path 7 we will look at habits and how they can be changed, so there will be much more advice about making changes stick then. But for now, well done – you have completed Path 1. I hope it has got you thinking and keen to move on to *Path 2 – Take personal responsibility*. I'll see you there on the next path.

Catherine's story

I first came across the *Positive Paths to Wellbeing* course at the start of lockdown. Like most people I had lots of time on my hands so it seemed like a great way to help me through those first few weeks, which at the time I did not expect to turn into months. What struck me most when I did the course was Path 1 – becoming really clear about what is important to me, which I had not given a lot of thought to. As I was entering my 40s it was becoming obvious that I needed to focus more on my physical health. I had been finding that I was much more affected by having an unhealthy day in terms of what I was eating, often feeling a bit lethargic. It became really clear to me that I needed to give more thought to what I was eating and when (no more late-night unhealthy snacks – well at least not so often), to getting the right type of exercise (I walk a lot but was missing out on strength training) and not drinking too much alcohol. I found that when I started doing some exercises first thing in the morning it really woke me up and meant I was much more focused on studying as I was also doing an Open University degree. I am happy to say that I just graduated. I do sometimes find that I have started to creep back to my old ways so I have revisited the paths on a few occasions to help me get back to a healthier way of life, which I know I prefer. Like everyone my life has its ups and downs but *Positive Paths to Wellbeing* helps me refocus.

Path 2
Take personal responsibility

'To reach a port we must sail, sail not tie at anchor,
sail not drift.' Franklin D. Roosevelt

2:A – Choose my response

In Path 1 we thought carefully about what is important to us and considered the past, the present and the future. I hope that you have started to think about some aspects of your life that you would like to change. And that is not because there is anything wrong with your current life, but it is about recognising that time never stands still and that life is constantly changing. Therefore it makes sense to think about the future, how things are likely to change, and to take control of how we want our life to develop and evolve. We might have a young family at the moment, but they will grow up and eventually move out. We might have a job that is satisfying now, but for how long? It's unlikely that it will be satisfying forever. I have had several careers (although I use the term 'career' loosely) as life simply does not stand still. Even if you are not for changing, everything around you is. Remember the days of having to queue at a phone box to make a call and push two-pence pieces into the slot – no? You are just a youngster then! Now we have a library, TV, phone box, bank, cinema, music venue and typewriter in our pockets. Times change and so do we. So Path 1 has woken us up to the thought of change, but we don't need to make any great plans yet until we have thought a bit more deeply.

I don't want you to feel overwhelmed either. There are so many opportunities available to us now. Not so long ago, certainly for my grandparents' generation, many people never even thought about leaving their home town, not even for a holiday. But now we can travel anywhere, move to a different city or country for work, take up jobs that did not exist 30 years ago, sign up for hobbies that we can learn about from our own living rooms and connect with people all over the world. So how do we find the time for all we want to do in this ultra-busy world of ours? We cannot do everything. I really want to emphasise here that *Positive Paths to Wellbeing* is not about being perfect. No one has ever been perfect and that even includes you and me. ☺ I don't want this book to put you under pressure to be perfect, to get everything right. That is simply not possible and it is important to acknowledge that. So relax, enjoy reading the book and when the time is right – you will know when that is as you will be itching to start – make your plans with the help of all the information you have yet to read. (Is that possible? Sounds like some sort of backwards time warp but I think you know what I mean!) This book is about working out what is right for you and helping you to focus on what is important in your life, helping you to find time for the things that make life happy, fulfilling, exciting and worthwhile.

Path 2 is about working out how you are going to get more of the important things into your life. And I'm afraid the only person who can do that is you – that is why it is called *Take personal responsibility*. Of course, you do that all the time now, but are there ways to think and act to make it easier? To make the good things more likely to happen?

The first milestone along this path is *Choose my response*. In Jack Canfield's book *The Success Principles*, he talks about how your response to an event determines the outcome.

Event + Response = Outcome

Let's say you are driving to work and there are roadworks and traffic jams. You are getting more and more stressed as you realise you will be late and you start shouting at the car in front, banging your hands on the steering wheel, your breathing becomes shallow, your adrenaline pumps up and you feel frustrated, angry and stressed. Eventually you arrive at the office, in a foul mood, late for work, the boss is angry and you can't think straight for an hour. So you make mistakes with your work and maybe mark yourself out as someone who is difficult to work with and moody.

Or, maybe you are driving to work and there are roadworks and traffic jams but you stay calm and ask yourself if there is anything you can do. Well, you can't get rid of the roadworks and traffic jams, but you can call the office and leave a message to let them know the situation. You can put your favourite music on or listen to an audio book. You eventually arrive at work late but ready to get going and everyone knows and understands the situation. You are your usual calm self, someone who is good to work with and reliable. So we have the same event but a different response and that gives us a different outcome.

Now take a moment or two to have a think about a difficult situation you have experienced recently. Break it down into *event*, *response* and *outcome*. Write down the event and your response and then the eventual outcome. Now think about whether you could have made a different response. What might have been the outcome? Obviously, you can only guess at that, but draw on your experience of similar situations.

Event: What happened?
Response: What did I do?
Outcome: What happened next?
What would have been a **better response**?
What might the **outcome** have been?

For me one of the most important ways I used this concept was as a parent.
Event: My 13-year-old daughter raises her voice to me about some rule I am imposing.
Response: I raise my voice back at her to emphasise my point.
Outcome: Spiral of shouting at each other and then afterwards I feel ashamed of myself – I am after all the adult! But I learnt a new approach.

Event: My 13-year-old daughter raises her voice to me – no change there.

Response: I stay calm and say something like, 'You sound cross and frustrated about this – tell me more.'

Outcome: My daughter calms down and we have a sensible, calm conversation.

Now this is not wishful thinking; this is what really happened. Once I started choosing a better response, we never shouted at each other again – and she is in her thirties now. By taking a very brief pause and engaging the thinking part of my brain, rather than the instinctive, primitive part of my brain, I was able to bring about a better outcome. And of course there are times when I still respond from my primitive brain – as I said no one is perfect – but by becoming more conscious that I do have a choice, I am more likely to be able to override a primitive response with a more considered one. Driver cutting me up at a junction: 'Please, do carry on, you must be in a hurry, I hope you get to the airport on time.' Waiter ignoring me or being brusque: 'They must be having a tough day, poor them.' Hanging on a phone for 40 minutes to a call centre: 'aaaaaggggggghhhhhh, just employ some more people you hopeless, incompetent company!!!!' Yes, we all lose it sometimes. But if we can lose it less with those people who mean the most to us, life will be on the up.

Sometimes when we think about the Event + Response = Outcome equation, we might only think of the 'response' as something we say, but it applies to any action or even inaction. Let's think about a few more examples.

Event: I put on 4lb after eating rather a lot of delicious jelly trifle over Christmas. Definitely one of my Christmas treats!

Response: I think I am never going to lose that weight now – at my age it is impossible to lose weight – so carry on eating unhealthy puddings each day.

Outcome: 4lb turns into 7lb which turns into a stone by the end of March.

Alternate response: It was only a Christmas indulgence, so get back on track with healthy eating. Have delicious natural yoghurt and fruit for pudding instead, with nutrient-packed nuts and seeds.

Alternate outcome: 4lb lost and back to pre-Christmas weight.

Or what if the response is a lack of action?

Event: My boss wants me to work late for the umpteenth time because they are disorganised and forgot to ask me to do something in a timely manner.

Response: Say nothing, work late, let a family member down who I was going to visit, then quietly fume.

Outcome: I miss seeing the family member and feel like a bit of a doormat for saying nothing, and next week exactly the same thing happens.

Alternate response: I explain to the boss that I have a commitment that evening and can't stay late but could do an extra 20 minutes. I ask if there is anything I can do to help make sure the jobs get to me earlier in the day.

Alternate outcome: Boss appreciates my help but knows they can't keep doing this and sets up a new system for handing jobs on. Or I discover the boss doesn't care about my life and I start looking for another job.

So what makes us respond in a way that is less helpful? Why don't we respond perfectly to every situation? Why not take a pause in your reading for a few minutes and have a think about why you and other people don't always choose the best response.

What did you come up with? It might be our upbringing – that is how our family behaved so we have learnt it from them. Yes, let's blame our family! Maybe we are tired or hungry and we respond in that way. Hangry anyone? (I no longer experience hangryness – you will find out my secret in Path 5). We might blame our genetics – we are all like that in our family. It might be years of experience when dealing with a particular person who pushes our buttons – we could call that an emotional trigger. Our environment plays a part – maybe we are in a situation that is stressful, such as the traffic jam. Maybe our hormones affect our behaviour – menstrual cycle and menopause for women, hormonal changes in young people, testosterone levels in men. Sometimes lifestyle can influence people – for example, when under the influence of alcohol and drugs. How about when we are ill or in pain? Don't we behave differently? Understandably. Age makes a difference – young people's brains are still developing. You may have heard of the amygdala, the primitive part of the brain that responds to emotion and is involved in triggering the fight, flight or freeze response.[1] The ability to override this emotional response is carried out by the pre-frontal cortex which does not fully mature until between about 23 to 25 years of age.[2] So young people have an excuse for responding more emotionally. That was what I came to recognise when I shouted at my daughter – I was the grown up, not her. I just wasn't behaving like one.

So the next time you feel an emotional response taking over, which might have an outcome that you don't want, try to engage the thinking part of your brain, your prefrontal cortex, and pause, breathe deeply, and choose a better response. I know it can be done as it transformed my relationship with my teenage daughter, now a wonderful grown-up woman. As I mentioned in the introduction, in *7 Habits* Covey talks about the space between the event and response. It is in that space that we have the power to choose our response. Sometimes the gap is just a fraction of a second, other times it could be minutes, hours or even days. If possible, actively taking a longer gap to think and consider our response can be very helpful. We won't always get it right – as I said it is not about being perfect because that is impossible, but just keep learning from experience. When I first came across this concept I did find that I was thinking a lot more, and choosing my responses more consciously. Obviously, I had been living on autopilot for some time!

When we look around us we can see examples of people choosing great responses and others who perhaps are not choosing so wisely. For me, there are some people I take inspiration from when it comes to choosing the best response. One of them is Jamie Andrew. He lost both his hands and feet following a climbing accident. But despite this he keeps finding ways to respond to all the challenges that life throws at him. He has run marathons, climbed the Matterhorn and developed a career as a motivational speaker, as well as being a dad to three children. When I find myself giving up easily with some new challenge I ask myself 'What would Jamie do?' and I know the answer – choose his response and find a way. Who do you admire and who motivates you when the going gets tough?

To summarise this milestone, we all have choices. Sometimes we respond out of habit or instinct and get an outcome we are not happy with, but we can choose our response, change what we say or do and achieve a better, more thoughtful outcome.

2:B – Focus on what I can control

The next milestone examines what is in our control and what is not. In 2:A we looked at our response to events and in this milestone we will be looking at the events themselves. If we go back to the traffic jam, we know that this event was not in our control. But how we responded to it was within our control. We might respond based on our primitive brain, or we might pause for a fraction of a second and respond more thoughtfully, from our higher brain. It helps to have this concept in mind when we are dealing with difficult situations.

I find that diagrams can help to illustrate a concept, so on page 31 you will find my 'circles of control' diagram. I first came across circles of control in *The 7 Habits of Highly Effective Teenagers*, by Sean Covey, when I was delivering a workshop, based on the book, to a group of school students.

Since I am still a bit of a teenager at heart, I really related to this simple concept, which looked at two areas – a circle of control and a circle of no control. But I do see a more nuanced halfway point – a circle of indirect control or influence. Maybe I am growing up after all! So let's examine my control diagram a bit more closely.

Circles of Control

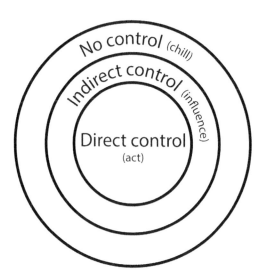

The central circle contains the things you have direct control over. Take a short pause and have a think about what you have direct control over.

Did you say your actions? The truth is that no one else makes words come out of our mouths, and no one moves our arms and legs about for us, so yes, our actions are in our control.

What about your thoughts? Do you ever have thoughts you don't want? I know I do. Things pop into our heads from seemingly nowhere, sometimes unwelcome. Of course there are many times when we choose our thoughts, for example when we are planning a holiday or working on a task. Or maybe you spend time thinking about the past, something that has happened either recently or maybe ages ago. But I don't believe we are in control of all of our thoughts. If you struggle with difficult thoughts and emotions there is a great book by Russ Harris called *The Happiness Trap* which explains a form of therapy called Acceptance and Commitment Therapy (ACT). In the book he provides techniques for managing difficult thoughts and emotions. I use techniques from this therapy with my coaching clients and find them to be very helpful. In Path 6 we will delve a little more deeply into a couple of these techniques. If you are finding that your thoughts are making life a struggle, please speak to your GP or a therapist. There are many ways to learn how to manage difficult thoughts and feelings, so don't try to face it alone – reach out for help. I will cover this more in Path 6.

Going back to the circles, we have direct control over our actions, although it might not always feel that way. As I mentioned before, no human is perfect, so you will never do everything right. Have you ever looked back on something you have done and wondered why on earth you did it? Yes, me too. Many, many times. So whilst we do have direct control over our actions, don't be hard on yourself when you get things wrong; that is normal. Just try to learn from the situation.

The middle circle focuses on indirect control. Have a think about what you have indirect control over. In other words, what does your behaviour influence? What impact do your actions have on others? How does it change the way they behave? So much of what we do affects others. As a parent I certainly had indirect control over my children. My example of shouting back at my daughter in the previous milestone is an example of indirect control. My behaviour influenced her behaviour. If you are a boss you can also understand that you have indirect control over your staff. What we say and do can heavily influence others. Think about how you would feel if you were having a good day and then you got an email from your boss criticising a piece of work you had just finished. Their behaviour (sending you the critically worded email) would have influenced how you felt and potentially how you responded. How would you have felt if the email was praising you for a great piece of work? It is clear that we are heavily influenced by the behaviour of others.

The outer circle looks at the things that you have no control over. Have a think about what might be in that circle.

What came to mind? The weather, the political situation, your age, your background and upbringing? The important message here is to recognise what is in our control and to let go of what we can't control, to focus on taking action where we can, but learning to 'just chill' if it is something we can't do anything about. I know that might sound rather flippant. I for one often worry about things that are out of my control. When we love and care for others that is not uncommon. I recall a time when my younger daughter was travelling from Australia back to the UK on her own while we remained in

Oz. The journey took almost 24 hours with a change of flight in Singapore and she was only 17 and off to start university. I think I worried and cried for the full 24 hours, while my husband, who is much better at chilling about things he can't control, just kept reassuring me that she would be fine. Of course she landed safely back in Scotland where her aunt was waiting to collect her. I was so relieved. So I know that chilling about the things that are out of our control is very much easier said than done, but definitely something to aim for, so that we can put our focus and energy into things we can control.

Now have a look at the list below and see where you think the items fit in the circles of control. Do they fit neatly into one circle or straddle two or maybe all three?

1. Delayed flight
2. My health
3. My past
4. How others treat me
5. Being late for a meeting

The answer often depends on the perspective you take and the circles can be a useful tool for helping to see things from different angles. Take the pandemic, for instance. Was it in our direct control? Absolutely not. For the first time in our lives we were ordered to stay at home, forbidden to leave the house except for essential food and exercise. It still feels fairly crazy when I think about it, but we complied in order to save lives. But were there some aspects that were in our direct control? Yes indeed. How I complied with these new rules was down to me. Whether I sanitised my hands, wore a mask, kept two metres away from everyone was down to me. Now, I am a rule follower so let me reassure you there was no Partygate in the Paterson household! And my behaviour would also have influenced others. Did anyone ask you to break the rules, such as pop into their house for a sneaky coffee? How you responded to that would have influenced them. But there was also so much that we had no control over – the virus for one thing, how the government responded and the rules it set out. I certainly tried not to worry too much, and to put the enforced 'stay-at-home' order to good use. I used this time to focus on getting my *Positive Paths to Wellbeing* course online and supporting others with their wellbeing. I did enjoy the change of life for a period of time although definitely got to the I-am-so-over-this stage eventually.

I hope you find this is a simple concept but also one that can be quite complex when you start to dig more deeply. And I hope you find it helpful. Going back to the earlier example of being stuck in a traffic jam, if I focus on what I can control I am more likely to make that phone call, listen to soothing music and calm my breathing rather than just getting all stressed.

2:C – Manage my time

So far we have thought about what is important to us (Path 1), and we are trying to focus on what we can control (2:B) and to choose our best response (2:A). Now we need to find the time to do the things that matter to us. There are so many books and workshops about time management and I have studied quite a few of them. In fact I ran workshops on time management when I worked in the NHS. So this milestone provides you with some top tips and techniques for getting more of those important things done.

The very first thing is deciding what is important. You simply cannot do all of the amazing things that are open to us in our digital, interconnected world. Hopefully you now have a better idea of what is important to you. I find it useful to picture a scale of importance with 100 at the top and 0 at the bottom.

Scale of Importance

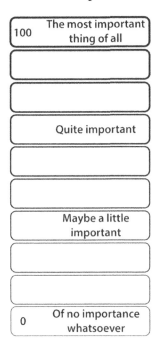

When you are trying to decide what to do with your time, you need to be focused on activities that are towards the top of the scale (100), and you need to say NO to those at the bottom (0). I know that is very obvious, but in reality we don't always do that. Come on, be honest – have you ever done a 'displacement activity'? You know the sort of thing. You have an essay to write or some life admin to do and suddenly tidying up a cupboard or watching Netflix seems like a much more tempting option. So this simple scale can help you prioritise. Ask yourself, on a scale of 0–100, how important is this? Now compare it to whatever other option is vying for your time. Filling in your tax return on 31st January – 95, watching *Game of Thrones* – 0. If you are already doing something important but something more important comes along, you have a way of assessing what you should do. Phone call from your child who needs help – 100. Even the tax return can wait under those circumstances.

You have probably heard of the story of the teacher who has an empty jar which they fill with large rocks and then they ask the class if the jar is full and the students say yes. The teacher pours in some pebbles and these fill the spaces between the rocks; the teacher asks again if the jar is full and the students say yes. Then the teacher pours in some sand which fills the spaces between the pebbles and asks if the jar is full. 'Yes!' cry the students. Finally the teacher pours in a cup of coffee and it fills the space between the grains of sand and the students laugh. The jar had not been full after all. The moral of this tale is the importance of filling your life with the important things, the large rocks, first. Your family, your health, your job. The things that, if they were taken away, would make life very tough. If you try and add them in after the less important stuff, the pebbles and sand, then there is no space left for the large rocks. One student asked what the significance of the coffee was. 'Well,' the teacher said, 'it goes to show that no matter how full life may be, there is always space for a cup of coffee with a friend.' Definitely a good maxim to live by.

So how do we get organised to ensure that the large rocks get done? In my time management workshops I share the acronym GOALS.

G = Goals
O = Organisation
A = Action
L = Learning
S = Self-awareness

Now let me take you through each of these five steps to help you make the best use of your time. This section will particularly apply to you if you work in an office environment, but it can also be relevant for other jobs or if you are retired and have a busy life, which of course many retirees do.

G is for Goals
It is first worth considering what makes us feel that we don't have enough time. Have a think about this for a few minutes and then look at the list.

- Lack of clarity about what is important in our life
- Thinking we can do it all (we can't)
- Perfectionism
- Difficulty prioritising
- Multitasking/switching
- Other people not being organised
- Distractions – people, internet, phones, etc.
- Not being good at saying no
- Procrastination
- Volume of work to be done at work and home
- Over-estimating what you will achieve in a given time
- Crisis management and firefighting, which is stressful
- Juggling caring commitments with work commitments
- Too many emails demanding attention at work

If we take number 1, lack of clarity, we need to return to *Path 1 – Clarify what is important to me*. As I said before we can't do everything that is available to us in this world, so setting some goals about what you want to achieve in the short-term and the long-term can be very helpful. Looking at the different areas of the Wheel of Wellbeing in Path 1 can also help to highlight the different areas of your life in which you would like to set some goals. You might be the sort of person who likes to look far ahead and have yearly goals, or that might fill you with horror because you prefer to be more spontaneous and not plan very much at all. And that is fine as we are all different, so decide what suits your personality best. However, whether you are spontaneous or planned you will still have goals that are aligned with your work, things you need to do. Plus, you will have goals linked with your home life. Determining what is right for you is very important as we are all different. No two people will have exactly the same work and home life, so don't compare yourself with others; work out what type of goals will be helpful for you.

We are much more likely to achieve our goals if we write them down. I love drawing out a mind map to provide a visual one-page reminder. We are even more likely to achieve our goals if we tell other people too. When I was writing this book I was making very slow progress but eventually got to the point when I really wanted to get it finished. I decided to announce it to all the people who had completed my *Positive Paths to Wellbeing* course, my alumni, as I call them. I also asked if anyone wanted to have a read through and hold me accountable for sending over a chapter a week. Thanks to my lovely volunteers, I started to make great progress with the writing as I had committed to getting it finished and I had told people! I did not want to let them down. But then some more important family issues came along and the book went on the back burner for a while, which was perfectly fine as I knew what was more important. You can see that the book eventually came off the back burner!

Another way to help keep on top of achieving your goals is to make use of technology such as tracker apps. If your goal is to run 5K and you have never run before, then using an app such as Couch to 5K can be very motivating, as can wearing a fitness tracker. Spreadsheets and charts can also be useful if, for example, you are saving up for something.

And don't forget that goals change as life happens, so don't be afraid to review your goals regularly and make adjustments. I mentioned in Path 1 not to make too many plans for change until you have finished the book, but just remember – if you do end up setting goals you can always come back and review this milestone.

O is for Organisation

If you know what you want to achieve it is helpful to be organised. David Allen in his book *Getting Things Done* uses the '4Ds' for time management, and I find this way of getting organised very helpful, especially for work situations.

The first D is 'do it now' if it takes less than two minutes. If it is a quick job that can be done in two minutes or less, it is much more efficient to just get on and do it. A good example is if you are looking at emails and a quick reply is all that is needed, then just get on with it. The exception is of course if it makes you angry – you know those emails – then pause and wait, maybe until the next day! The same goes for texts.

The second D is 'delete it'. If it isn't for you, just delete it, get rid of it – you don't need it cluttering up your life. Or if it is a physical object such as some junk mail, throw it away (or preferably recycle it).

The third D is 'delegate it'. Can you get someone else to do it? Is there someone else who ought to do it or who would benefit from doing it, perhaps because they get to learn some new knowledge or skill?

The fourth D is 'defer it'. In other words, do it later. For this you need a good system to capture all your deferred actions. So let me go through the elements of a good system.

Firstly, I need to say that you must find the right way to make this work for you. Some people like everything to be electronic and accessible on their phone, whilst others prefer paper systems or maybe a mixture of both. I am firmly in the camp of using a mix of electronic and paper systems. There are lots of apps that can help you get more organised so you will need to investigate them and find what works best for you. This section is really about the principles of a good system, and exactly how you organise it will be down to your personal preference. I don't think I have ever seen two people's systems looking exactly the same.

Components of a good system
1. Diary/calendar
2. Notes
3. Projects
4. To-do list
5. Waiting
6. Reading
7. Contacts
8. Files
9. Checklists
10. Time-saving technology
11. Emails

1. Diary/calendar
So the first thing is a diary or calendar. As I said this can be paper or electronic. This is where you record all of your appointments and commitments, and you should also use it to plan what I call 'time with myself'. This is where you book

out time to be focused on something that is important for you to do, such as writing a report or setting aside time for life admin or going for a walk or to an exercise class.

You should also use your diary to mark in things you need to do on a specific day, such as checking someone has got back to you or to download boarding passes for a flight for example. If you only use a paper diary you can take photos of the pages when you add something in. This acts as a backup, in case you lose it. I am a bit 'belt and braces' here as I love my paper diary but I also add everything into my electronic calendar on Outlook too.

2. Notes

You need somewhere to write any notes that you want to make as you go about your work. It is best not to write on lots of little scraps of paper as you will only lose them. With a notebook you can always go back and find what you were looking for.

3. Projects

In the front of my notebook I have a list of all the projects I am involved in. David Allen calls anything with more than one action a 'project', so we are not just talking here about big things such as planning a wedding, which will have hundreds of actions, but we are also talking about small things like booking a holiday, which might only have about five actions. I find my projects list very helpful as a memory jogger and for longer-term planning.

4. To-do list

You also need a to-do list. I have my project list at the front of my notebook and my to-do list at the back. A to-do list must only have single actions on it. So, for example, 'organise a conference' is a project but 'phone hotel to book venue' is an action and should be on the to-do list. If you prefer an electronic option, you can use tasks in your email account for your to-dos or a reminder list on your phone. There are also project management apps you can use to manage all of your projects and your to-dos. Do get into the habit of writing down everything you have agreed to do on your to-do list immediately. Otherwise you will forget some things and maybe get known for being unreliable. If you have everything captured in a good, reliable system, David Allen assures us we will have more space in our brains for interesting, creative thoughts. How about that for a bonus? I really think it is true. If you are spending lots of your brain power thinking, 'Don't forget the…' (whatever it might be), you don't have space for exciting and interesting planning and problem solving.

5. Waiting

You also need to keep track of things you are waiting for. I have a few ways of doing this. I don't cross off actions on my to-do list when I am waiting to hear back from people, but instead I put a star in the margin. You can also have a waiting folder in your email account to keep track of people you are waiting to hear back from. This is very important as it can feel very satisfying to cross something off your to-do list because you have emailed someone, but if it is just as important to get a response back from them you need to keep track of it. Otherwise it might be the sort of thing that can wake you up in the night – 'Oh no, I did not hear back from Bob and now that report needs to be in tomorrow and I forgot all about it!'

6. Reading

You need a way to keep up to date with articles you want to read. This might be setting up a special folder in your email or having a box for hard copies. Keeping on top of your subject is very important for your career, so having reading material to hand when you are filling dead space, such as waiting for a meeting to start or travelling by train, is a good use of time. I keep podcasts and audio books relevant to my business for when I am driving and doing the ironing. It makes both tedious jobs zip along much more pleasantly.

7. Contacts

You need a good contacts list. This is so much easier with mobile phones, but make sure you update contact details as soon as someone sends you new information. This is an example of a quick two-minute job, so do it straightaway. You don't want to waste time hunting for that new phone number you remember seeing three weeks ago.

8. Files

Filing is important. Make sure your electronic files are stored in such a way as to be backed up. You can back up on an external hard drive, or on the cloud or at work in shared folders on a server. Maybe even all three! Never trust anything to only your computer's hard drive. You have been warned! I recently heard of someone who had hundreds of files on their computer when it died and they lost everything. Don't let it happen to you, but if it does, go to an expert computer shop just in case they can recover anything. I hate losing a few paragraphs, so I don't know how I would cope with losing all my files!

Old-fashioned paper filing is reducing rapidly as offices and homes become more paper-light. I follow Marie Kondo's advice (the Marie of *The Life-changing Magic of Tidying* fame). Because we don't receive so much paper through the post for life admin anymore, I have a plastic wallet in the kitchen and I put all of the paperwork into that folder. I set up a new one each year. I have only used one folder per year since starting this four years ago. If I do need to find a document it does not take long to go through the folder, and it is much less tedious to chuck everything into the folder than to file it away in a filing cabinet, which I never did, instead I had random piles of paper around the house. If you do have lots of paperwork this might not work for you, and it certainly won't work in many office settings, but I am sure you already have a decent paper filing system at work, as you will have been doing that for years.

9. *Checklists*

Speaking of things you have been doing for years, do you have tasks that are repeated regularly? I have run workshops for years, and for these I have a checklist so that I don't forget anything. If you do a regular task, then a checklist is invaluable. I was shown the importance of checklists when I worked in the health service as the use of checklists for patients in Intensive Care brought ventilator-acquired pneumonias down to very low levels.[3] After this great improvement, more and more routine procedures had checklists developed to ensure all staff followed the best procedure each and every time. They don't have to be complex. Often the best checklist is only a few items long, but getting it right every time can be so important, even lifesaving. I have a Christmas checklist and a holiday packing checklist, so they can be for fun stuff too.

10. Time-saving technology

What about all the time-saving technology we now have? Everything from shopping and banking apps to password managers to voice-activated digital assistants ('Hello, Alexa'), and where would we be without Google Maps? Lost! Artificial intelligence such as ChatGPT and others are changing the way we work and live. It is an exciting time. It may take a bit of effort to learn something new, but if it is useful in the long run it will have been worth it. Just make sure the tech doesn't actually use up more time than it saves, or it is a false economy.

11. Emails

Now let us turn our attention to the dreaded emails. There are two main schools of thought when it comes to emails: either let them pile up and don't worry about organising them, an approach I use for my Gmail account, or keep on top of them and be organised. For my work emails I tend towards a more organised system, which is a version of Inbox

Zero. You will find lots of information about it on the internet. If you aren't happy with how your emails are organised and they are causing you stress, have a read of the next section and see what you think. I know many people who have adopted this system and prefer it as they feel more in control. For Inbox Zero you set up folders with the following labels.

@Action
@Waiting
@Reading

I have an extra one called @Maybe for things I might one day have time for but are not a current priority. (That day has yet to come!) By putting the @ sign at the front, it moves these folders to the top of your folder list. Then when you sit down to look at your emails you apply the 4Ds that we talked about earlier in this milestone.

If an email only requires a quick reply (less than two minutes), apply the first D – do it now. So many emails just take a few seconds to reply to. Remember not to reply quickly if the email has made you angry or upset – we have all had some of those in our time. If it is something you have replied to, but you need to hear back from the person, move it to the @Waiting folder.

If the email is of no importance, apply the second D – delete it.

If someone else is more suitable to deal with the email, apply the third D – delegate it – by forwarding it to them. 'I wish I had someone to pass things on to,' I hear you say!

If it requires some action, apply the fourth D – defer it – and move it to the @Action folder. If it is something you want to read, move it to the @Reading folder. If you want to keep it, but it does not require any action, move it to one of your other folders for filing.

In this way, when you sit down to go through your emails, your aim is to clear your inbox. Hence the name Inbox Zero. Then when you have time to deal with the tasks you have deferred you will work from your @Action folder. But don't feel all smug when your inbox is empty; don't forget what is waiting for you to attend to in the @Action folder. I find that I sometimes forget to look in my @Action folder, so I also write any actions on my to-do list, but then not being a digital native, I think my brain defaults to the low-tech solutions first. Periodically you will want to check your @Waiting folder too, to see who you need to chase.

I find this system works really well for my work emails, but for my Gmail account, which has all the usual subscriptions and the daily deluge of random emails, I adopt a different system called Inbox Infinity. I don't bother with clearing it out or filing emails unless something is very important, so I just let it build up, and if I need something I just search for it. I do have plans to delete the emails in my Gmail account, as the storage of data uses energy in massive data centres and is not a very environmentally friendly option. So do think carefully about the data you need to keep and try to delete unnecessary emails and documents.

So there are different options depending on what works for you. You might want to get sophisticated and use more of the tools that your email provider supplies, so why not take a course or have a search on the internet for some tips on making the most of your email system. I have just covered some basic principles here, but I am most definitely not someone who uses all the aspects of Outlook, despite having taken a course a number of years ago. The fancy search and flag functions never really stuck for me, but Inbox Zero has stuck for many years, so it works with my brain. You need to find what works for you.

Are you someone who stops what you are doing every time you hear the ping that lets you know an email has arrived? Yes, I must confess that is often what I do. The allure of finding out if something interesting has arrived in my inbox, especially if it is an enquiry from a potential new client, is very addictive. There are times when that is just fine, but if I need to do a concentrated piece of work I make sure my email is off and I only check it when it is ok to take a break. There is still the danger of getting side-tracked, but if I stick to the discipline of doing the most important things first, unless the email seems even more important, I try to leave it until I have more time to devote to answering emails. And using an out-of-office reply can be helpful for setting other people's expectations about when they might hear back from you and takes the pressure off you to respond to emails quickly. You don't only have to use out-of-office for holidays.

Your mobile phone also has an allure all of its own, so being disciplined when you are doing an important piece of work and putting your phone away in a drawer or even another room is good practice. You can also download an app[4] to stop you using it. A number of years ago I worked on a project with families and one of the biggest problems was the use of phones by the children – something that has got even worse. The families were having so many arguments about mobile phone use and I thought that what is needed is a phone prison. I thought 'tech time out' would be a cool name. A box that could be set with a timer so that the box would stay locked for a certain amount of time that you could select. All the parents agreed that it would be a great idea and I even went so far as to look into the manufacture of such a thing, as I could not find one on the market. I discovered that there was a patent on a timed locking box in America so I abandoned the idea of going into full-scale manufacture, but I was sure it was a winner. So I was delighted to discover such a thing existed a few years ago and one of my coaching clients, who was a student, bought one to help him be disciplined as he wrote up his final year thesis. It really worked for him and I loved when he took ages to reply to my messages because his phone was in his 'phone prison'. Definitely something to consider if you are too tempted by your phone and easily distracted. It might be something you could use with children who find it hard to stop checking their phones. Put all the family phones in for a few hours and find something non-digital to do instead. We all need a helping hand when it comes to willpower. I certainly know that I do. We will look at willpower in more detail in Path 7.

A is for Action
Now that you know your goals and you are organised, you need to take action. So what are some of the top tips for getting things done?

Schedule

Scheduling the day can be very helpful. Breaking it up into sections can help to reduce overwhelm and keep you focused on the task in hand. I have a daily planner/journal that gets me organised first thing. At the top of each page there is a section to complete on what I am grateful for. It is a lovely way to start the day, and expressing gratitude has been shown to help with mental wellbeing.[5]

Prioritise

My next task is to list the most important actions that I need to get done that day. These are the three or four key things from my to-do list that I've prioritised; if I get them done that day and nothing else, it will have been a good day. I prioritise them with a number and I try to stick to that fairly strictly. Those are definitely the days I am the most efficient. Brian Tracy, author of *Eat that Frog* advocates doing the hardest thing first. Get it over and done with and then that glow of satisfaction and achievement will lift you up. I can't say I always follow this advice, but I am certainly always conscious of it and try not to leave the more difficult things until later in the day when my energy will be much lower. Don't forget to look ahead when selecting your actions for the day – look to next week, next month or later in the year. Sometimes we put things off that are not urgent, but if we leave them long enough they do become urgent and cause us stress, so be organised and plan ahead.

My daily planner has space for my appointments and I also note down what I am going to do for my physical and mental health. These of course are high priority and we will look at them in detail in Paths 5 and 6. I also wonder what challenges I might have during the day and how I might solve them. And, no, I don't have a crystal ball in my office, but I do find it very helpful to have a think about potential challenges so I can plan ahead. I had a look back at the last few months in my planner/journal to see what I had written in answer to that question and one of them was 'focus on the book; it is more important than tidying'. I think I must have been doing some displacement activities instead of writing this book. And, hey, having identified that challenge a few months ago is probably one of the reasons that you now have the book in your hand. I pre-empted my tendency to procrastinate over a hard task by spending some time at the start of the day examining the potential challenges. So having a rough idea of how your day is going to pan out and what you are going to be doing is very helpful. It is important to be flexible with this too because we rarely know exactly how long something will take and who knows what more important thing might turn up and take us away from our plans. If you are interested in purchasing a copy of my planner/journal to help keep you on track every day, you can find it on Amazon.

Make tasks smaller

One of the reasons we put off the hard tasks is that they can feel overwhelming. Just too difficult! But if you can break the task down into smaller chunks, it might be easier to tackle. What is that old joke – how do you eat an elephant? One bite at a time. So the next time a task feels overwhelming, see what smaller stages it can be divided into, and consider what is the next step you can take to move it forward.

Let's take doing a spring clean as an example. (Does anyone actually do that any more? But you know what I mean.) One of your rooms has turned into a junk room and the thought of clearing it out is too much. So you chuck something else in and close the door. Well, that is what sometimes happens in my house! But just doing one shelf at a time or seeing what you can manage in 10 minutes can be very helpful for getting started. And that is another great tip that I often use – what I call 'jump in for 10'. I just do something for 10 minutes that I have been putting off, and if I want to stop after 10 minutes that is just fine. There are some tasks that once started must be finished, but for many things 10 minutes will make a difference – and you never know, you might do a bit, or a lot, more.

Focus

Sometimes I need the exact opposite of that tip, and that's when the 'exam' technique is useful. If I have a piece of work that I really need to get done but have been procrastinating over, then I approach it like an exam. Turning off all distractions and setting aside a few hours to power through it can mean I achieve a first draft. I then feel so much better now that this task that has been niggling at me, or even worse, stressing me out, is nearly complete. Sure, I will need to give it an edit, and that may take longer than the draft, but the feeling of relief is wonderful.

Take a break

Having said all that, it is not a great idea to be sitting at your desk for hours on end so you might want to try the 'Pomodoro' technique. You may well have heard of it. Work for 25 minutes, have a 5-minute break and then repeat. You can get Pomodoro timers for your desktop or your phone, and the idea is to complete three or four Pomodoros and then take a longer break. You decide what works best for you. Oh, and make sure you get up from your desk during the break and have a stretch.

These tips can also apply to non-writing tasks such as housework. Do a housework exam or gardening Pomodoros.

Reduce time wasters

All these tips are based on us being paragons of virtue who are focused all day long, but do you have any time wasters? What are the things that suck you in and before you know it an hour has gone past and you are down the rabbit hole of cute kitten videos or endless Instagram scrolling. Or you just veg out on the sofa and watch some TV. Yes, me too! Some of these things are great for a bit of relaxation but it's not so good when they become excessive. So know what wastes your time and work out how to limit these things. The wide range of activities we can access in the comfort of our homes is rather addictive and it is very easy to keep going back for more. There are no easy answers to this, but developing some practices and rules around it can help. There are some apps[4] you can download to block your phone for a set time, so you might want to try those out. Or maybe you will buy a phone prison like I mentioned earlier. Or you might create some guidelines around when you can watch TV and record things that are on outwith these times.

I don't want to demonise phone use or TV watching, and I do love both, but just check that the amount you do provides good relaxation and is not eating into time that would better serve your physical and mental health. I do think that the advent of phones has encouraged us to multitask, to switch between different tasks rather than concentrating on one activity alone. I know I might have the TV on and be scrolling through my phone at the same time. I have found that taking up knitting has cut this down. You can't knit and scroll at the same time!

Don't multi-task

Now I want you to do a little exercise. I want you to write the following and time yourself. And, yes, you will probably need to get your phone out for the timer and then you are going to hop on to your emails or social media of choice so maybe you will come back to the book another time.

Ah, you are back! Great. I want you to write 'I am a good multitasker' followed by the numbers 1–19 underneath as shown below. Do it as quickly as you can and time yourself.

I am a good multitasker
1 2 3 4 5 6 7 8 9 10 11 12 13 14 15 16 17 18 19

Now I want you to do a second exercise. This time you are going to write the same sentence and set of numbers but start by writing the first letter, then the first number, then the second letter, then the second number and so on until the sentence and numbers are complete. So you will write *I* then *1*, *a* then *2*, *m* then *3*, *a* then *4*, *g* then *5* and so on until the two lines are complete. Again, I want you to time yourself.

So how did you find that? Did you take longer the second time? Did you find it harder? This is a simple example of how multitasking is not the best option.[6,7] It is better to focus on one thing at a time, because it takes time and energy for our brains to keep switching back and forth between one activity and another. This is why we are more efficient when we focus on one task and really get into what is called 'flow' or 'being in the zone'. So the next time you have something important to do, try to eliminate distractions, turn your phone off, gather everything you need to get the job done and keep focused. You may even find you enjoy it.

Batch tasks

Batching tasks is another great way to keep your focus on one area. It is often much more efficient to wait until you have a similar group of tasks to carry out and then to power through them in one go. Have a think about some small tasks that you do that might be better done in one longer session. This applies to work and home tasks. For me, in my work, there are various websites that I use that require small inputs. If possible I try to do a number of them at the same time rather than opening up the website, inputting one set of details, then switching to another task. Domestic duties such as ironing lend themselves to batching rather than setting up the ironing board each day for your work clothes. Batch cooking is also very popular and you can find videos on the internet to inspire you.

L is for Learning

So you know your goals, you are organised, and you are taking action, but what if you are still struggling to manage your time well and to get things done? Maybe there are things you still need to learn, to allow you to make progress. When I find that I am struggling to do something, I ask myself if it is because the task is beyond my current knowledge and skills. That is often, even usually, the case.

When I started my business there was so much to learn that I did not have a clue about. Video-editing, learning platforms, bookkeeping – oh goodness, the list goes on and on and on and on. I soon discovered that when I was procrastinating it was because I did not really know how to do something. Maybe I had a vague idea, and indeed a little knowledge can be a dangerous thing. If I needed to write something in a foreign language, say Spanish, then I would not have a clue and so it would be very clear that this was not a job for me and that I would need to get help. But when you have a vague understanding of something you often think you can do it, but the very thought can be overwhelming. If it is something that you really have to do yourself then you will need to learn more about it. The great thing is that there is so much information available on the internet, so chances are you will be able to access some learning without too much difficulty. But if it is something that will take too long to learn, or something that you won't need to use very often, then you are usually better off finding someone with the skills you need. Time is money, as is often quoted, so be pragmatic and seek help. We all need it sometimes. We will look again at learning in more detail in Path 8.

S is for Self-awareness

Managing our time well is often down to our own self-awareness. If you know your goals, are well organised, are taking action and learning what you need to know, there may still be barriers to achieving your goals and getting things done. Let me take you through a few common ones.

Generally we need to be self-motivated. Our drive to achieve something is best if it comes from a desire inside of us rather than being externally imposed. So if your work life does not spark any self-motivation, it might be an indicator that you are not in the right job. And if you are lacking motivation and it is linked to feeling 'tired all the time', as many people are, then taking better care of your physical and mental health can help you to re-discover your energy levels and self-motivation. We will cover this in Paths 5 and 6.

For many people perfectionism can get in the way of getting anything finished, and if this applies to you then seek out some support to help you set the right standards, so you are getting things done that are good enough. Never be afraid to ask for help. You may need to choose wisely who you ask, but there are many people willing to help, so seek them out.

One of the main reasons we can feel so busy is because we say 'yes' to things we should say 'no' to. I am sure you have experienced that inner sinking feeling when you have agreed to do something you would rather say no to. Because you have clarified what is important to you in Path 1, you should have an idea of your main priorities and you can use these to help you find a way to say no, albeit politely. Here are a few possible replies.

- I'm afraid that I don't have the time to do that right now.
- I can't help with that right now, but I might have time next week.
- I can't help with that, but I know that Jane is great at that; why don't you ask her?
- I'd love to help but I have to leave at 5pm today.
- My priority now is X, so I am unable to commit to Y.

A clear **no** is far better than a **yes** that you don't deliver on. No one benefits then. And remember, everything that you say no to, gives your time for something positive to say yes to.

I hope that working through the five areas covered in GOALS has helped you think about getting more organised and managing your time better. You will discover more tips in *Path 7 – Develop positive habits*, when we look at willpower, but for now take some time to think about whether there is anything in this milestone, *Manage my time*, that you would like to implement.

Gill's story

I found the information in Path 2 very beneficial for me at work. Work is always very busy, and at times I felt overwhelmed by the sheer quantity of emails I received each day. I just never felt I was on top of them, and consequently I worried that I had missed something important. When I did the *Positive Paths to Wellbeing* course and Marie explained the concept of Inbox Zero, I thought I would give it a go! I set up the necessary folders and soon found that I had a system for reading and filing my emails. It really helped me to get organised and to feel on top of my work. There are still some days when I am not as organised as I would like to be, but I now have the structure and routine that I need and I can quickly get back on track.

I have also found the advice to 'just do 10 minutes' has been great for helping me to learn a bit of Spanish. I had been going to lessons, but then was unable to attend for a while. I thought I would get really behind but decided to focus on what I could control and to use a language app each day instead. It meant I managed to keep my hand in whilst not being able to commit to the lessons. I then didn't feel that I was too far behind the other students when I was able to get back to the lessons and was still confident to try out a little on holiday. Small steps really do add up!

Path 3
Nurture my relationships

'The only way to have a friend is to be one.'
Ralph Waldo Emerson

3:A – Nurture my relationships with others

During Paths 1 and 2 we have mainly focused on looking at ourselves: what is important to us and how we can ensure we get those important things into our lives. Now we are going to consider our relationships with others. Humans are social beings. We need other people, although maybe not all of the time. I don't know about you, but I certainly need some time on my own on a regular basis, but I also need the company of others. If we consider that solitary confinement has been used as a punishment, it is clear that being with other people is important – definitely something worth remembering if you ever wish everyone would just go away!

The first thing I would like you to do is to make a list of all the different roles you have in your life. For example, you might be a partner, a parent, a child, a sibling, an uncle, a neighbour and a friend. You might have some work roles:

your professional role with clients and customers for example, or you might be a colleague or the boss or an employee. If you were a teacher you would have a role in relation to your students. And maybe you are active in your community. Do you have a voluntary role or are you part of an organisation such as a church or club? Have a good think about all of the roles in your life. I have provided a list for you below, but I am sure you can think of more.

- Partner
- Parent
- Child
- Sibling
- Grandparent
- Grandchild
- Aunt/Uncle
- In-law
- Cousin
- Friend
- Neighbour
- Volunteer
- Club member
- Worker (e.g. teacher)
- Boss
- Employee
- Colleague
- Student

Now I want you to choose some of the most important roles and imagine you are at a party where the person you have this relationship with is going to make a speech about you. Maybe for a special birthday with a zero at the end, or perhaps a leaving do at work. Whatever you are imagining, make sure you are the centre of attention. Now what would you like that person to stand up and say about you? Not what **would** they say, but what would you **like** them to say? If you really don't like the idea of being the centre of attention, then just imagine what you would like them to think about you. Spend a few minutes writing a short speech about the type of person you want to be for this important person in your life. If you are thinking about the role of parent, what would you want your child to say about you, or what about your partner, your friend, your boss or your client?

This is not an easy exercise to do at first and it might feel awkward thinking about what you want people to say about you, but it gives you some very valuable insights into the type of relationships you want to nurture. You might want to start with a role from your home life and then follow that with a work role. You may want to revisit this exercise later for some of your other roles. Pick the most important ones in your life to start off with.

How did you find that? Probably quite difficult. I know because I have used this exercise with many people. But did you also get some insights? I remember one of my clients, on completing this exercise, saying, 'I don't know how my wife puts up with me!' He said it slightly jokingly, but it was a profound insight, which made him determined to make some changes in his relationship.

Now I want you to go through these imagined speeches, and score yourself out of 10 on how close you are to that being true right now. If you think, 'Yes, that is how our relationship is right now,' then score yourself a 10, but if you are some way off, then the score will be lower. You might want to speak to the person who is in that relationship with you, but you don't have to; it can be a private exercise that you keep to yourself. The choice is yours. If you have some relationship speeches where your score is low, have a think about what you can do to bring the score closer to 10.

Let me give you an example. When I did this exercise many years ago, I asked myself what I would want my children to say about me at a big birthday speech. The two main things that came up for me were that I wanted them to say that Mum made time for us and that we had fun. So I made a determined effort to be more available and to try to be more fun. I did a bit less housework so that I had more time for them. Children aren't usually too bothered about a tidy house! I certainly never achieved a 10, but I was much more conscious of the time I spent with them and my attitude to life generally.

So spend some time thinking about a few small things that you can do to move your scores closer to 10. Write them down. As before, don't make plans for great big changes as chances are they will overwhelm you and will soon be forgotten. Try out small changes – they can have quite an impact.

One way of looking at nurturing your relationships is using the analogy of maintaining a house. In order to have a nice house to live in, you need to look after it. You need to wash the dishes, sweep the floor, tidy up. In the longer term you need to paint the windows, clean the gutters and wash the patio. A house needs regular small amounts of nurturing and so does a relationship. And occasionally it will need a larger piece of work too.

Relationship building   **Relationship damaging**

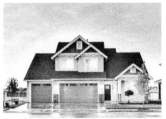
(B Mellish from Pexels)

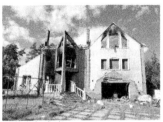
(Y Sukhenko from Pexels)

So what are the things that nurture relationships? Think about the little things that you do or say in your everyday interactions that build the relationship. Obviously, these things will vary depending on the relationship you are thinking about. If you think about the role of being a parent, what nurtures that relationship? It might be spending time with your child, listening to them, comforting them, reading with them. You will also need to set boundaries and enforce them. It is important to realise that nurturing a relationship is not just about being 'nice'. Sometimes it is about doing the harder things, like saying no when your child wants to take their phone to bed to text their friends in the middle of the night!

And what about honesty or 'diplomatic honesty' as I prefer to think of it? This is a term I heard that I thought perfectly describes the need for honesty, but not brutal honesty, which can be harsh and painful to hear. We do spend most of our lives being diplomatically honest. We don't say exactly what is in our mind when invited to a relative's party that we know from experience will be a bit hard work. (Just being clear in case any of my relatives are reading this: that does not apply to you!) Maybe we say we would be delighted to come along, and we make the most of the party as it is important to us to be supportive of our relatives. We are not being brutally honest, but diplomatically honest, in order to preserve the relationship.

I remember working with someone who had a difficult relationship with their stepson. This man had a tendency to be brutally honest, telling the child that he found him difficult. The stepfather felt it was wrong to pretend otherwise. But he did desperately want to have a good relationship, as he saw the stepson regularly and loved his stepson's mother. Pretending to like the child under these circumstances was a relationship-building action, even though it did not feel completely honest. Brutal honesty was a relationship-damaging action. Over time, the stepfather used diplomatic honesty more and more often, and reduced the brutal honesty. As a consequence their relationship improved and he came to like his stepson more and more. You may have heard the phrase 'fake it till you make it'. If the underlying reason why you are faking it is honest and good, then this can be a good strategy for building relationships. Over time your feelings can change because you are behaving more positively to the other person, and they in turn start to feel more positive towards you. Remember the circles of control from Path 2? Our behaviour affects the behaviour of others, as we have indirect control or influence over them. I am sure you can imagine how the stepson behaved when his stepfather told him he did not like him.

What about at work? Again, many of the same behaviours that nurture your home relationships will nurture your work relationships. You may also have some behaviours that are particular to the culture of your work which may not apply in a different workplace.

So take a bit of time to think about your different roles at work and at home, and write down the behaviours that build up that relationship. I have given a few here, but I am sure you can add in others that apply specifically to your roles.

Relationship building actions

- Listening
- Saying thank you
- Spending time
- Having fun
- Being patient
- Praising
- Using diplomatic honesty
- Helping
- Keeping promises
- Cuddling
- Being non-judgemental
- Being kind
- Setting boundaries
- Keeping calm
- Providing support
- Being positive
- Showing empathy
- Showing love
- Being intimate
- Showing interest
- Caring
- Forgiving
- Being consistent
- Being punctual

If we now consider what damages a relationship, we can continue with the analogy of the house. The house could be damaged purely by neglect, or it could be something even worse – such as active destruction. I am fascinated by a house near where I live that was only built about 15 years ago but has been so neglected that it now looks very dilapidated. The window frames are rotting, the garden is overgrown and there are plants growing out of the gutters. Neglecting a relationship can be damaging too. And it could be even worse with someone actively breaking the windows and knocking down walls. So what neglects or damages relationships? You can probably list the opposite of the behaviours above, but there are other actions that can be damaging too.

With a child it might be criticism for something they have little control over, such as how quickly they learn to read compared to their brother, or maybe telling them they are useless when they have struggled with an activity. I often find I notice parents being harshly critical of their children when I am in the supermarket. I have sympathy with the parents who are feeling frazzled, but I have more sympathy with the children who are just being children! How we talk to children is so important for their development, and focusing on relationship-building actions and reducing relationship-damaging actions is vitally important.

It is not just children we can get into bad habits with and find that relationship-damaging actions become the norm. With a partner it might be constantly criticising them and not noticing all the little things they do to make your life easier. At work it might be micro-managing a member of staff rather than giving them proper training and then some autonomy to get on with their work. Now take a few minutes to think about your relationships and what behaviours damage them. Do you agree with my list below?

Relationship damaging actions

- Criticising harshly
- Criticising the person not the action
- Breaking promises
- Embarrassing them in front of others
- Being cruel
- Being impatient
- Being negative
- Making unreasonable demands
- Not allowing them to be themselves
- Ignoring
- Judging
- Taking credit for others' work
- Being unreliable
- Being selfish
- Belittling
- Being lazy
- Being unfair

I am sure you can add more if you think about your different work and home roles. Again, I want to emphasise here that this is not about being perfect. You are not going to magically turn into a saint and never do anything to damage a relationship. This is not going to happen, because all sorts of situations influence our behaviour, as we spoke about in milestone *2:A Choose my response*. It is about becoming more aware of the actions that build and the actions that damage, and trying to tip the balance in favour of the positive actions. It is also worth knowing that what is a building action for one person can be a damaging action for someone else, or at the very least a fairly neutral action. Let's say you have two children who are very different from each other, as most siblings are. For one, going to the park to play football could be a great way to spend time together, but the other one might hate that. For them, going to the cinema or spending time crafting together might be an activity they would love to do with you. Your building-and-damaging-actions lists will vary depending on the relationship you are considering. So now why not choose a relationship that could do with a bit of nurturing and then focus on saying and doing things that nurture and build up this relationship? Really try hard to avoid, or at least reduce, the words and actions that damage the relationship.

One way that I used this concept was with my then teenage children. I realised that I had been doing a lot more of the damaging behaviours. You maybe know the type of thing: 'Come on get up! Why do I have to keep calling you?' or 'Why aren't you eating your breakfast? I have spent ages preparing that for you – how ungrateful.' Then when they came home from school: 'What are you doing dropping your bag there? Don't you think I have anything better to do than to pick up after you?' or 'You are not going out looking like that are you? You look a fright!' or 'In my day…' Ok, I hope I never said that last bit, but you get the picture. (Incidentally, when I have shared that confession with workshop participants I have often been asked if I've bugged their house! So it is a very familiar behaviour.) Once I became more conscious of my behaviour I vowed to focus on relationship-building behaviours and to reduce the damaging ones, and it really brought about a change in my relationship with my teenage children. There was less tension and more fun, and home became a happier place to be.

In my workshops when we explore this concept, the talk sometimes turns to destructive relationships, where someone seems to be actively causing damage to the relationship. The need to set boundaries, and if necessary excluding the person from the relationship, is so important. A relationship needs to be good for both parties involved. If not, it can never be a healthy relationship in the long term. This is not something I am covering in this book, but if you need support to leave an unhealthy relationship, seek out help. There are public services and charities[1] that can help.

I hope that the concept of relationship-building and relationship-damaging actions has been helpful and that you are nurturing your relationship houses! Our relationships are one of the most important things for our overall wellbeing. Before you go on to the next milestone, why not spend a few minutes thinking about some small actions you can take to nurture the relationship with someone important in your life, where the relationship is not as good as you would like it to be. You might be surprised by how quickly the relationship can change.

3:B – Nurture my relationship with myself

We have spent some time thinking about our relationships with others and how we can build up those relationships. For this next milestone we are going to think about our relationship with ourselves. Does that seem like a strange thing for me to say – your relationship with yourself? We do have thoughts and feelings about ourselves just like we have thoughts and feelings about others. And we can improve this most vital of relationships just like we can improve our relationships with others. After all, who do we spend the most time with? I don't know about you, but I can't ever seem to get away from me – she follows me everywhere!

You might want to think of nurturing your relationship with yourself as 'self-care'. Caring for yourself. Knowing what makes you feel good, improves your wellbeing and lifts you up. And reducing things that damage your sense of wellbeing, make you feel bad and bring you down. Now this whole book is very much about looking at all the different aspects of your life that impact on how you feel about yourself, and feeling good about ourselves is something I am sure we would all like. As we explore the different paths on the journey through the book, you will identify many ways to improve your wellbeing, but for now just make a few notes in answer to the following questions.

1. What improves how I feel about myself?
2. When am I at my happiest?
3. When have I been my healthiest?
4. What fills me with excitement?
5. What is most challenging in my life?
6. How do I look after myself?
7. What are my strengths?

I hope you have paused and taken a few minutes to answer the questions. Remember you won't have been to Peru if you only read the guidebook. Did you get any insights as you answered those questions? Maybe some of them were difficult to answer. If you found 'what are my strengths' a tricky one, maybe you are a bit hard on yourself and rather modest. The culture you were brought up in might be one where you were criticised for being proud of your skills and achievements. 'Getting too big for your boots' or 'blowing your own trumpet' might have been considered bad character traits. But has this made you overly harsh about your own abilities and achievements? No one is listening, so have a go at listing all of the things you are good at. Be proud of what you have achieved. Think about your home life and work achievements, your schooling, your sporting or musical talents. Maybe your best talent is being kind to your elderly neighbour, or remembering birthdays and making people feel special. Maybe you are always at work on time and work hard, or you can be relied on to help your friend with her children after school. Don't be shy; make a long list.

Now you might have started to have a niggly thought: 'Yes, I might do that, but my colleague Maggie is so talented; she has a busy job, two children, plays the violin and got awarded an OBE!' We so often find that we compare ourselves to others unfavourably. Maybe you think a colleague is smarter or a friend is more successful, or a family member is more likeable than you will ever be. But comparing ourselves to others is not very helpful if it lowers our self-esteem and prevents us living our lives the way we want. After all, we are all absolutely unique individuals, so comparing ourselves to others is natural, but not necessarily helpful. No one has had exactly the same life history as you, so how can you really compare yourself with others?

The next time you find yourself being self-critical, ask yourself this: what would my best friend say? I bet you have often comforted someone who was being too tough on themselves and said something like 'but you are a great colleague' or 'you're such a supportive friend – don't be too hard on yourself'. And that is exactly what I want you to do for yourself. Be your own best friend. Be a realistic critic, not a harsh one. Be a support, not a judge. Try and see if your own inner best friend can stop criticising you but instead ask what you can learn from this situation. It is not about being accepting of low standards, or poor behaviour, but about recognising that we are only human, that we do make mistakes and that we can't be good at everything. So take a pause and answer the questions below.

1. When do you compare yourself to others?
2. In what ways are you more critical of yourself than of others?
3. How do you feel about the concept of being your own best friend?
4. How can you be more compassionate to yourself?
5. What can you do to nurture your relationship with yourself?

Let us all try to be more compassionate towards ourselves as well as others. Wouldn't that make the world a better place?

Before we leave this section, see if you can take some time over the next few days to add to your answers and develop a deeper insight into what you need to do to care for yourself, improve your wellbeing and improve your relationship with yourself. When you understand more about what lifts you up, you can start to build more of those life-affirming times into your daily life. They can be very small things, like taking a few deep breaths, or actions that take more effort, such as learning a new skill. Or maybe it is about having different thoughts and being your own best friend more often. Whatever they are, becoming more aware of them will help you to include them in your life and nurture your relationship with yourself.

Another important thing to remember is that often we feel guilty about looking after and taking time for ourselves, but it is important to care for yourself. Otherwise eventually you won't be able to care for the important people in your life if you get physically or mentally unwell. It is like the warning on the plane – put your mask on first so that you can then help others.

Maria's story

My relationships with my family and friends have always been really important to me, but Path 3 gave me another way to look at my relationships. I loved the concept of the relationship house: how important it is to give time and thought to developing relationships and how they can deteriorate through damaging acts or even just neglect. I became more conscious of keeping up the important connections in my life. I make sure I organise regular catch ups with my family and friends. I try to be a good neighbour and pop round to visit, especially if I know there has been a happy or sad occasion. I love doing small acts of kindness including sending my partner messages during the day to thank him for something he has done. This path really showed me the importance of people in my life. I know that when I do something for someone else's good, I also feel good too. Everyone wins! I also don't forget to nurture the relationship with myself and I make time for activities that lift me up, such as regular exercise and time alone. I have loved all of the *Positive Paths to Wellbeing* course and it has been a great help in keeping me positive during a time of major change.

Path 4
Improve communication

'The single biggest problem in communication is the illusion that it has happened.' George Bernard Shaw

4:A – Recognise we are all different

In Path 3 we started to think about our relationships with others and we are now going to spend a bit of time thinking about how we communicate with the people in our lives. Improving communication is a great way to nurture our relationships.

Now I don't know if you share one of my traits, but I am aware that I don't like it when people disagree with me. When they see things differently from my viewpoint. I sort of bristle with the need to emphasise my point and I don't really take their point of view or opinion as seriously as my own. Since becoming aware of this tendency I am working hard to overcome this and to embrace other people's views, but it is still a work in progress, and I honestly think it always will be. I think it stems from my dislike of arguments and conflict. I so often hear people say that they don't like conflict, and I am certainly one of those people, but it is not healthy either to suppress your own opinions or not to welcome the opinions of others, so this is definitely something to work on if you feel the same way. Now of course I know there are some people who love a good argument and are just delighted when people disagree with them so they can have a really interesting, and maybe even heated, discussion. This is just one simple example of how we differ in our personalities. So have a think about how you feel when people don't agree with you. Do you take it in your stride and embrace the different opinions, or are you more like me and find it difficult?

So why are we humans so different? Well to start with we have different genetic codes that we are born with, then we go on to have different upbringings and life experiences. We may well have siblings, but even though we may have been brought up in the same family we will have experienced different schooling, different friends and even different attitudes from the same parents. Looking at our present-day, grown-up lives, no one else has the same life as you. You are influenced all day long by the interactions you have with the people around you and the world you live in. It is therefore not at all surprising that we see things from our own perspective, and through our own experiences, which is why we so often disagree with each other. And this can be made even worse if we don't take the time to look at things from the other person's perspective and try to understand their point of view.

Many years ago I trained as a mediator so that I could help to resolve disputes between staff. This was usually when the relationship between two members of staff had completely broken down. Mediating was not an easy task, and it was one that I most definitely needed training for if I was going to have any hope of making things better rather than worse. What made me realise that I needed training was that on one particular day I had been asked to 'facilitate' a conversation between a manager and their member of staff, where the relationship was rather tense to say the least. It had got to the stage where the staff member had been moved to a different site to keep the peace. As I had 'facilitator' in my job title I was picked as just the person for the job. However, I soon came to realise that this role required skills that I did not possess. All was going well, and they had listened to each other and apologised, but then the manager asked the member of staff to return to their old place of work and the member of staff point blank refused. I was completely stumped as to what to say next as they both looked at me expectantly and my brain froze; I thought, 'S*&t! I have absolutely no idea what to do now that is not going to set us back to square one or worse.' Fortunately, thanks to my forward-thinking boss, I was soon able to get trained as a mediator, and I came to realise that the main role of a mediator is to help people to see other perspectives rather than only thinking about their own. Then they are less likely to dig their heels in and refuse to co-operate, especially if they have been helped to see the longer-term consequences of their actions. Ultimately a mediator aims to help the people involved to come to a resolution that will work for both sides.

You might think you always see both sides of a disagreement because you see things from a factual basis rather than from your own perspective, but there are a number of experiments that have shown that we screen out a lot of information. I remember attending a conference where they showed a video and asked us to watch out for changes to the background, and then afterwards they asked how many changes we had seen. I was watching very intently and managed to spot about three. The actual answer was over 20. I felt rather embarrassed at my lack of observation skills, but most other people had only seen a few changes too, so it wasn't just me. I have since used that video in my own training and have had participants who did not spot any changes at all. That was a very effective way of showing me and the participants that we are not always right, that we do not in fact take in everything that is going on around us. Of course intellectually I knew that already, but did I really believe it? I thought if I was looking at something and it changed, I would notice it. But I had not noticed very much at all, even when I was staring at it. That simple exercise at the conference really changed my perspective and made me question myself more – in a good way. You can search for selective attention tests on YouTube and see how you get on. It might surprise you too.

Now I want you to have a think about a relationship where you and another person don't always see eye to eye. Maybe you regularly disagree with that person. Please spend a few minutes thinking about your different backgrounds and how that has shaped the people you are now. If you think about the different backgrounds of a parent and child, or a boss and their employee, it is a wonder that we ever see eye to eye at all.

Think about what gets in the way of good communication between you and this person. Can you start to understand why they have different views and opinions from you? How can you try to understand them better? Also have a think about how you can help them to understand you better too. After all, communication is a two-way street.

When you think about a parent/child relationship and the different eras they were born and brought up in, it is far easier to see why there are differences of opinion. I was brought up in a different country from my parents. My mother grew up on a small farm in rural Ireland and I was brought up in inner city London. Such a contrast between the two. So we definitely did not always agree on everything and, with the benefit of hindsight and maturity, I can see why. Now I can see the positives. I love going to Ireland to visit my family now that they have returned to their homeland. I love the Irish culture and I am proud to have Irish ancestry. Being different adds interest to life, so we really should embrace and celebrate it.

Once you have thought about why you are so different from that person you don't always see eye to eye with, can you come up with some ideas for improving the relationship? You might want to look back at the list of relationship-nurturing ideas from Path 3. You may well have many work relationships where your backgrounds and life experiences are completely different. Maybe your colleague comes from a different country or has a different ethnic or religious background. When I worked in the NHS I was a member of a group that looked at how the services we provided were experienced by different people based on the protected characteristics set out in the Equality Act 2010 (UK). The protected characteristics are listed below.

1. Age
2. Disability
3. Gender reassignment
4. Marriage & civil partnership
5. Pregnancy & maternity
6. Race
7. Religion or belief
8. Sex
9. Sexual orientation

It was very helpful to consider how the services the NHS provided were experienced by people from each of these groups. Members of the public were part of the group so they were able to bring different perspectives to the discussions. Having someone who is blind provide feedback on how difficult it was to attend appointments made me more aware of my limited viewpoint as an able-bodied, middle-aged woman. Looking at access to services from an age perspective was also very important as, fairly obviously, it is older people who use the NHS most, but how easy is it for them to get information, especially in an increasingly technological environment? What about if they are not very mobile – how easy is it for them to access a health centre or hospital? How did staff address people who had same-sex partners? Was an assumption made about the gender of their loved one? Or what about patients who had a religion that affected their choice of food or other considerations?

Navigating difference is not easy, and there is a lot to consider, but it is crucially important in understanding each other. It is so important to recognise that not everyone is like me and to really embrace and celebrate differences. How dull would our world be if we were all the same? If we liked exactly the same things and agreed on everything, life would be very limited. So the next time you find yourself feeling irritated that someone sees things differently from you, remember that we are all different and accept that we all see things differently and that this enriches our lives.

4:B – Focus on a deeper understanding

Path 4 is all about improving communication, and in this milestone we are going to look at how to get to a deeper understanding of other people. One of the problems is that people often don't really listen to each other. Have you ever noticed that? Someone interrupts the person who is talking when they are just a few words into what they want to say. How can they have listened and understood before they formulated their reply if they have only heard a few words? Do you recognise this scenario? I know that I do as I am one of the people doing the interrupting! Yes, that is another of my not-so-good habits. But I am trying hard to be a better listener. In *The 7 Habits of Highly Effective People*, Stephen R Covey used the phrase 'listen with the intent to reply' and I have to admit that really did apply to me and it frequently still does. For a better understanding Covey says we need to 'listen with the intent to understand'. So how do we do that? Well, improving our listening skills is one way, and in this next milestone we will consider a few different listening styles.

Before we do that, can you spend a few minutes thinking about how good you are at listening? Think about how you are with different people. You might be a good listener at work but not so good at home, or vice versa. Take a few minutes to pause and answer these questions.

1. What do you do well?
2. What would you like to improve?
3. Do you listen with the intent to reply or the intent to understand?

Don't ignore!

Now we are going to consider some different common listening scenarios. First, think about a situation where you have not been fully focused on the person who was talking to you. Maybe it was a child who you were ignoring because you were busy doing something else and did not have the time (or maybe the inclination) to listen to them. I vividly remember doing this when my children were young, and I did not have the patience to listen to all of their chatter. I am sure that is something played out in houses all over the world. Realistically, I could not have given them my full undivided attention at all times, as like all parents I had jobs to do in the house while taking care of them. But did I listen attentively to them at the right times? I am pretty sure the answer is no.

Maybe you have a colleague in the office who would happily talk all day long and you would get the sack if you paid rapt attention to every word they said. And increasingly in our modern world I see families out together at a restaurant and they are all looking at their phones rather than paying any attention to each other. What does this do to family relationships and the ability of children to develop good conversation skills? And how do you feel if you are being ignored when you want to speak to someone? Frustrated? Cross? Like you are not important?

Now we obviously cannot listen attentively all day long, and there are times when we might legitimately only half listen, such as when your child is chatting endlessly or that colleague is continually talking, but we do need to make sure that we don't ignore people when they are feeling emotional; whether that is happy, excited, angry or sad, and they are needing our attention. Making a concerted effort to focus on the other person is a great way to nurture our relationship with that person, which will reap rewards both now and in the future.

Don't make it about you!

Another type of listening you may have experienced is when the other person is attentive, but they take over and make it all about them. Have you ever started telling someone about a holiday you have just booked to Spain and before you know it, they are telling you all about the holidays they have had there and what they enjoyed the most? Or you are excited to share a promotion you have received at work, and they immediately tell you about the promotion they received that was bigger and better than yours. I am sure most of us have experienced a version of this when our conversation gets hijacked. Do your conversations sometimes get taken over by others? Or maybe you are the one who takes over and you do the hijacking. I have found when discussing this in workshops over the years that there are people who recognise themselves instantly as those who take over and other people who would never dream of doing that. So which camp do you fall into? I must confess to being one of those people who takes over! But I am much more conscious of it now and hope that I do it less often. I find myself trying to rein back when I realise what I am doing.

Now, this type of take-over conversation is not always inappropriate, and it does happen naturally in social situations. I am sure you can recall sitting with a group of friends and someone starts off a topic and then others join in with their experiences. That is all fine and part of the to-ing and fro-ing of social conversation, but it is important to be aware of giving people the space to talk, especially when they are feeling emotional, whether that emotion is excitement, anger or maybe sadness.

Good listening

What makes for good listening when it is really important to listen well, such as when the other person is feeling emotional? First you need to allow the person to complete what they want to say without interrupting. Then, to get to a deeper understanding, you can ask for more information about any part of the story that does not seem clear to you. You want to get a full picture of the situation. You may know about the use of open and closed questions. If you ask open questions, where the answer needs to be detailed rather than a simple one-word answer such as yes/no, then this can help to convey that you are interested in the person and want to hear what they have to say. If you are not sure how to frame an open question, a simple option is to say, 'Tell me more about...' When I am coaching, I try to use open questions as much as possible so that the client can think more deeply about the issue we are discussing. Simple examples are: how did that make you feel, what ideas have you had, what options have you considered? With all of these I am avoiding telling the person what to do. Why is that so important, as surely we are having the conversation so that I can impart my 'amazing wisdom' ☺ to my client? Now sometimes people will want your advice, but it is best to wait to be asked. And, of course, you may have a job where people go to you for advice and are expecting to receive some guidance. But most of the time, with friends and family, when people are emotional they just want to be listened to. They don't want your advice, or if they do they will ask for it.

I remember a time when one of my daughters was upset as she was so busy with an exam coming up, a driving test on the horizon and some other stresses in her life. She came to speak to me and I gave lots of advice: 'Why don't you do this?' and 'Why don't you do that...?' You know the sort of thing. Well she went away more upset than when she had come to see me. I was annoyed with myself for forgetting all my training on effective listening so I called her back, held her hand and bit my tongue. 'Tell me more' was all I said. She started to talk through all that was worrying her and came up with a number of ways she could sort out the demands, and she went off feeling much better and with a clear plan of action that was hers and not mine. One of the most important things I have learnt over the years as a mediator and a coach is that people need to find their own solutions.

Now spend a few minutes answering the listening questions below and have a think about whether you need to make some changes to your listening skills. Don't forget that this is not about being perfect. If you are naturally chatty and tend to dive into conversations, you will no doubt find it difficult to change, but do your best to listen carefully when someone is feeling emotional and needs you to listen. And when you are having a light-hearted chat over a cup of coffee, don't worry about it so much – enjoy the banter! And what about if your phone is a major distraction? Try to have phone-free time to concentrate on your family, friends and colleagues.

1. How good are you at listening at work?
2. How good are you at listening at home?
3. As a listener, what do you do well?
4. Do you listen with the 'intent to reply' or the 'intent to understand'?
5. Are you often distracted when someone is talking to you, e.g. when using your phone or watching TV?
6. Do you tend to take over a conversation and make it more about you?
7. Do you tend to give advice even if it is not asked for?
8. What aspect of your listening would you like to improve?
9. Who do you need to listen to in a better way?

To summarise:

- Focus on the person and not yourself, and don't be distracted by your phone or anything else.
- Don't interrupt and take over. Don't make it about you.
- Don't give advice unless you are asked for it.

Written communication

Now it might seem like this is all one way. You might be wondering – when do I get listened to in all of this? In the next milestone of Path 4 we will look at how you can get your side heard too as we explore how to resolve conflicts. But before we go on to that I want to take a while to consider written communication. So far we have been focusing on spoken interactions, but for very many people a large part of communication at home and work is written, either by email or text.

When someone reads an email or text message they may not interpret it in the way you intended. Have you ever been involved in a misunderstanding over text or email? The recipient took offence or was upset at the content or tone of the message, when the person sending it did not mean to cause any upset. This can lead to considerable difficulties with a cost in time, energy and emotion to find a resolution. It can even damage relationships permanently. So, if possible, only use email and text for non-emotional topics and pick up the phone, video call or meet the person face to face if you think the conversation could cause an emotional response. In my experience this is more likely to lead to a quick and satisfactory conclusion than by exchanging endless angry or upset messages. But what if it does lead to a conflict situation?

Read on for the third and final milestone of Path 4 as we look at how to resolve conflicts.

4:C – Resolve conflicts

The third milestone of Path 4 is all about resolving conflict, and it applies equally to more minor disagreements or differences. As I mentioned previously, I trained as a mediator and have carried out many mediations with staff who have been in conflict. When I took them through the mediation process they almost always reached some sort of solution. But one of the saddest things to me was the fact that their dispute had reached the stage of needing mediation. Most people are simply not trained during their education to resolve conflicts. If we were all better equipped with these skills we could sort problems out as and when they happen and not let them escalate, and then a lot of heartache could be avoided.

The method I am going to explain to you is based on my experience of working with people in conflict and is drawn from a number of resources that influenced my mediation style. I was heavily influenced by the work of leading mediators Fischer and Ury and their book *Getting to Yes*. Stephen R Covey's *The 7 Habits of Highly Effective People* has a focus on working well together, which also shaped my style, and I received fantastic training from Core Solutions in Edinburgh. This is the method I found to be most helpful over many mediations.

If we look at the diagram below, we can think of the problem in the middle and the two people in conflict on either side, each with their own preferred, but opposing, solution, indicated by X and Y. Typically they battle it out until eventually the stronger one wins and their relationship is badly damaged, potentially forever. A better way to resolve this conflict is to be on the same side, working together, and coming up with lots of new ideas to potentially resolve the issue, indicated by ideas A, B, C and D in the diagram.

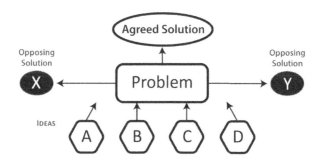

Now take a minute to think about any situations you have been in recently where there has been conflict or disagreement. This might have been with a family member or a work colleague, and then please take a few moments to answer the questions below.

1. How did the situation make you feel?
2. How did it get resolved?
3. Did you come to a solution or agreement you were both happy with?
4. What lasting impact did the disagreement have (if any)?

If when you think back you realise that the situation could have been handled better, let me take you through a six-step process that might make it easier for you to deal with disagreements or conflicts in the future.

1.   Check willingness to find a solution

Resolving any conflict is only possible if the other person is willing to work with you on it. Most people are reasonable and don't want difficulties to persist, so hopefully they will respond positively to a request to 'sort this out'. That phrase might come across as quite aggressive so it is best to start off with a kinder, gentler request. Maybe say, 'I don't know if it is the same for you, but I would really like to find a way to solve this disagreement we are having and in a way that works for both of us.' You are immediately making it clear that you want a solution that works for both of you, which is really the only way that you will get the best outcome. Obviously getting a solution that works for both sides is not always possible, but it is important to start out with that intention. They may want to set up a time to discuss it rather than talk about it at that moment, but that obviously depends on who the disagreement is with. At home you would probably talk about the issue there and then, but in a work setting you might arrange a meeting for a later date.

What happens if they don't want to play ball and have a conversation? That is when it gets a bit tougher! It is worth spending a bit of time thinking about the consequences of not talking and asking yourself the following question: what do I think might happen next if we don't talk? Think through all the possible scenarios that might play out. Then maybe you can find another way to approach the person and persuade them to talk. Whatever happens, you don't want the dispute to escalate and get even worse, so it is vital to spend time imagining all the possible likely scenarios so you can make an informed decision about your next course of action. You may then decide to involve others to try to resolve it such as a manager at work or for more serious issues a lawyer. Sometimes you will conclude that on this occasion you will do nothing and that might be the best option, although a hard one to accept.

2.   Listen without interrupting

The next step is to ensure a complete understanding of the situation on both sides. To do this, one of you needs to start first and explain your side of the issue without interruptions from the other person. It is not always easy to have a conversation about a disagreement without interruptions, so it is best to let the other person speak first and tell them that you won't interrupt. Now this might seem like a strange thing to say to them, but it sets an expectation of how you want to be listened to and shows respect for the person speaking too. Imagine this in a parent/child disagreement – how often do we let them speak without interrupting? Not very often if my experience is anything to go by. But that just might be me!

3.   Check you have both understood the issue

The third step is for the listener to check they have understood what has been said. So many times in a mediation when I asked the listener to repeat what they had heard, the speaker said, 'That is not what I meant.' We might speak the same language, but we often only hear from our own perspective. You then need to swap over so that the speaker becomes the listener, and the listener becomes the speaker.

4. Look for further information to explore deeper reasons behind the conflict

Sometimes people don't divulge the full story or their deeper motivations, so it is always worth asking if there are any further reasons why someone feels the way they do or has made the decision they have made. In this way you will often find out more and get to a deeper and more complete understanding of each other's position.

Sometimes it does not matter how much people talk as they will never agree to see things from the other person's perspective, and then it can seem like a solution is not possible. But all is not lost. If you do keep arguing backwards and forwards and blaming each other for the situation, then you can still acknowledge that you are not able to agree on this matter but agree to draw a line under it and move on to the next step.

5. Develop new solutions

This involves being creative and coming up with as many different solutions to the problem as possible (i.e. A, B, C and D in the diagram), even if some of them seem crazy. Sometimes crazy ideas spark off new thoughts that can lead to a creative, workable solution.

If your dispute is with someone like your boss it can be difficult to make the suggestion to look for new solutions, as you may expect them to take the lead in resolving the dispute. It is still worth being a bit brave and asking if together you can think of alternative options, as almost everyone is happier if problems are resolved quickly and without wasting valuable time and generating a lot of unhappiness. This step is much easier if you are the person in the position of greater authority or you both have equal authority. Then it is time for the final step.

6.   *Evaluate the ideas and agree next steps*

You may have come up with a few ideas and it may not be immediately obvious if all or indeed any of them will work, so you may need to go away and evaluate whether any of the ideas are viable. You will then need to agree a time to meet again and feedback your findings. Then you can plan how to move forward and to put your disagreement behind you.

Hopefully you can see that this is a useful process to go through which can help you reach agreement. Sometimes it can be helpful to have a third party who has been trained in dealing with conflict to guide people through the process, but most of us are perfectly capable of sorting out disagreements ourselves, with a bit of careful planning. I have helped many people have this type of conversation and they have almost always reached an agreement at the end.

Now please spend a few minutes answering the following questions on resolving conflicts.

1.   What are your thoughts on the six-step process?
2.   How would you describe your usual conflict-resolution style?

3. Thinking back to the earlier questions about a conflict or disagreement you had recently, could you have applied this six-step approach in that conflict?
4. In what relationships do you think you might find this process useful and why?
5. In what relationships do you think it would not work and why?

Let's work through the process with a hypothetical situation where you want to have Fridays off and so does your colleague, but one of you has to be in the office on a Friday each week. Your colleague (who is of course being unreasonable) says it is much more important for them to get Fridays off as they have children to look after, and yours are grown up.

You start with asking if they will have a chat with you about it so that you can find a solution that works for both of you. Reluctantly they agree! You ask them to start first with explaining their situation and state that you won't interrupt. They explain that their children finish school at 12:30pm on a Friday and they don't have any childcare in the afternoon. You summarise what they have said and make sure you have got everything right. You explain that you have an art class you want to sign up for on a Friday afternoon and it does not run at any other time. You say, 'Can I check you have understood my situation?' and they summarise what you have said. You ask, 'Is there anything else I should know about the Friday situation?' and your colleague explains that they are struggling to pay for any extra childcare, and it is really essential for them to have that time off. You add that you have been on a waiting list for this art class for two years and now that you have a place, you don't want to let it go.

It seems an insurmountable problem, until you explore Step 5, which is to think of any new solutions together.

1. Let the boss decide who works Friday – one of you may 'win' but you have little control over the decision.
2. Work alternate weeks.
3. Your colleague finds someone to help with childcare.
4. You find a different art class.
5. See if anyone else can help out with a rota for the Friday.
6. Ask the boss if you can trial closing the office on Friday afternoon.
7. Consider the longer term and find a new job with Fridays off.

You discuss the options and if necessary go away and find out more and then meet again for a further discussion. Maybe you will need to compromise and work alternate Fridays. Or maybe you do come up with other options such as agreeing to work more Fridays during the school holidays when the art class does not run, and your colleague finds someone to help out during term time, but then has more Fridays off during the holidays.

What happens if you still can't reach an agreement? It is very important to think about this possibility and what might happen as a result, and then to explore those potential outcomes too. In this scenario, you might need to let your boss or the Human Resources (HR) department decide and neither of you may get Friday off. Or your relationship might be strained and affect every day, not just Fridays. It is important to spend time thinking about what might happen if you can't come up with a solution together. A jointly negotiated agreement has got to be better than an acrimonious dispute involving your boss and HR.

If you find yourself in a situation where you want to use this process, you will almost certainly feel anxious and nervous about it, and that is only to be expected. But don't let that put you off trying to find a good solution. You can explain how the six-step process works in advance, and give the other person time to think about it before sitting down to discuss the situation. In that way they won't be feeling surprised, and possibly threatened, by the process.

This type of process doesn't just fit the workplace – what about with teenagers? How much better is it to sit down and calmly talk through issues and come to a joint agreement than it is to argue, or maybe not talk at all, and then have rules imposed that make the teenager resentful? The teenager is then more likely to want to exert their control by disobeying. I know which option I would choose.

I hope these three milestones – recognising we are all different, focusing on a deeper understanding and resolving conflicts – will help you improve communication with those important people in your life.

Grant's story

I studied the *Positive Paths to Wellbeing* course and found that a combination of *2:A Choose my response* and *4:B Focus on a deeper understanding*, really got me thinking. I realised that when I was asked a question, both at work and at home, I would provide a quick response that was based on my perspective – my thoughts, my ideas and mostly my needs. I often made statements without necessarily thinking about the other person's perspective. Once I started learning about these concepts in the course, I started to think more about the role of the other person in the conversation. What did they need? Why were they asking? What thought processes might they be having? I stopped answering 'straight from the hip', which I tended to do, and I became more thoughtful. At least I think I did – maybe you should ask my family and colleagues about that! I also recognised that good leaders answer with questions rather than statements. In my work role I have always strived to be a good leader, but this change of thinking has made me more approachable and tangibly more relaxed. It reminds me of my younger self too, the way I was when I was 25! The modern workplace, with its increased diversity and flexible working, is far better suited to this more considerate leadership style. I do still sometimes forget and fire off a quick response, but I then realise this, pull myself up, choose my response and focus on a deeper understanding. I'm told by those around me that there is a positive difference.

Path 5
Look after my body

*'Take care of your body – it is the only place
you have to live.' Jim Rohn*

5:A – Eat healthily

Paths 3 and 4 have focused on our relationships with others and now we are going to return to thinking about ourselves and specifically our body, or our physical health. We know that feeling good physically impacts on our overall wellbeing, and three important factors that affect our physical health are nutrition, our level of activity and how we sleep. So the first section of Path 5 is all about eating healthily.

One of the most frustrating things about trying to work out what constitutes a good diet is that we keep getting conflicting messages. For example, we are told that something is bad for us, then it is good for us, then bad again. A food movement starts that is anti-carbohydrate and then we read an article in the paper about how bread is good for us. We have pro-meat diets and, in contrast, the vegan diet.

It is so hard to know what to eat for the best! So why don't the experts agree on what we should be eating? One of the reasons is that nutrition studies are still a relatively new science and also it is very difficult to do controlled trials on humans when it comes to food. We have to accept that nutrition studies are an evolving science and focus more on what the majority of studies agree on, as well as what works for us as individuals with our different genetic and cultural backgrounds.

I have completed a nutrition coaching certificate so have been steeped in the science and the psychology of helping people to eat more healthily. This part of the book is based on my studies, and on reading many books and articles with different viewpoints on healthy eating. I am not a dietician or nutritionist; this section is based on my interest in the role of food in overall wellbeing, so please read my thoughts on nutrition with that in mind. If you have specific issues which you feel a change in nutrition would help with, please seek the appropriate expert guidance.

What I am going to share with you are a few simple guidelines and I want you to consider whether they work for the unique person that is you. Many hundreds of books have been written on nutrition, so this short section is going to give you my take on healthy eating – please do think critically about the following information and do your own checking if there are things I say that you disagree with. A book on wellbeing would not be complete without some thoughts on healthy eating, so I hope the rest of this section gives you food for thought whilst acknowledging that information about nutrition is always changing and that different experts have different opinions based on the complexity of researching human beings!

Reduce ultra-processed foods

One of the easiest rules to follow for healthy eating is to eat fewer ultra-processed foods.[1] Eat more foods that are largely unchanged from how they are found in nature. If a food has been through many processes in a factory, try to avoid those. It is such a simple rule to follow and one which can make a really big difference. This advice fits well with the diet that has the most evidence for being healthy, the Mediterranean-style diet. It comprises vegetables, fruits, nuts, herbs, spices, beans and other legumes, fish, seafood, wholegrains and extra-virgin olive oil, plus low amounts of meat and good quality dairy such as natural yoghurt and cheese. You can see that none of these are ultra-processed foods. You can adopt the principles of this diet but choose the types of vegetables, fruit, fish, etc, and how you cook these foods to suit your own culture. Trying to eat locally grown and seasonal food is also good for you and good for the planet.

So let's compare a few ultra-processed foods with whole foods. First thing in the morning, especially if you are in a hurry, you might opt for a breakfast cereal biscuit. When I read the label of a well-known version I saw that it had 20 ingredients, including some you would never find in a home kitchen. Now compare that to a whole food alternative that our grandparents would recognise – porridge – which has one ingredient. You know which one I would opt for.

Another option you might have for breakfast might be an egg, with some tomatoes and mushrooms – again single, unprocessed ingredients. And what if you wanted some toast with your egg? In this case try to buy the best bread you can afford, maybe from a local bakery, and try to have wholegrain rather than white bread. Or why not make some bread yourself? It is not too difficult, but it is very satisfying. What would you spread on your toast? Well, again, if we use the principle of single ingredients, butter would be my choice rather than a heavily processed margarine, but this is one area where you will still see differences of opinion on which is better for you. The debate stems from butter being higher in saturated fats than plant-based margarines. While there is still some debate on whether saturated fats are bad for you, the predominant view is that they are linked with heart disease (although this is disputed by some nutrition experts). On balance, for now I am eating butter in preference to margarine, but I use it sparingly.

I like some jam occasionally, so I buy a jam that is just made from fruit and fruit juice with no added sugar. This is following the principle of finding the least processed option. So in trying to reduce the amount of ultra-processed food in your diet, it is helpful to think about how to make your current food choices better. Some nutritionists would suggest I should avoid jam completely as it is high in sugar, but I prefer to adopt a more liberal approach as I believe that prohibiting things completely can make us crave them even more. I make sure my diet consists mainly of the healthiest options and I enjoy less-healthy food too, just less frequently.

Obviously if food is in short supply for any reason, we wouldn't have the luxury of turning down any food at all. And many people are in this situation. I certainly don't believe in demonising any foods, but where we do have a choice, then thinking in terms of 'basic' and 'better' can be helpful. So, the cereal biscuits in the example above are 'basic' – you wouldn't turn them down if you had nothing else to eat – but homemade oatcakes are 'better'. Orange juice is basic, because all of the fibre and many of the nutrients have been removed and it is high in sugar, therefore an orange plus a glass of water is a better alternative. For dinner a ready-meal lasagne would be basic; a home-cooked version is better.

We so often hear about junk foods, which are foods that are high in saturated fat, sugar and salt with little nutritional value, but often very tasty! If you think about a burger, 'basic' might be one from a fast-food takeaway; 'better' might be a burger from the local butcher, served in a roll from a local bakery, with lots of salad and some home-cooked potato wedges.

If you only follow one principle for healthy eating, then this is the one to follow: eat minimally processed food or process it yourself. In other words – cook! And if you can do this most of the time, you can't go far wrong. You will naturally increase the fibre content of your diet, reduce the sugar and salt content and increase the nutrients. Spend a few minutes thinking about a typical day's diet and identify any ultra-processed or factory-made foods you eat. Then try to think of a better, less-processed alternative.

Increase vegetables
Another important element of healthy eating, that is generally agreed on by the nutrition community, is that non-starchy vegetables should make up a large portion of your

diet. Lunch is a good meal to start packing them in. For example, homemade vegetable soup or a delicious salad with lots of different plant ingredients would provide a good healthy lunch, maybe with some homemade oatcakes plus houmous or fish to provide some carbohydrate, protein and fat.

Increasingly I am seeing advice that half of each meal should be non-starchy vegetables. That might seem like a lot of vegetables, but it is something to work towards. Even adding one extra veg to each meal can also make a difference and might be an easier way to think about improving your diet. Or maybe you could have a side salad with dinner? And you may also have heard the phrase 'eat the rainbow'. All it means is getting a wide variety of different coloured vegetables so that you are eating a diverse range of health-giving nutrients.

Fibre, prebiotics and probiotics

Eating plenty of vegetables (including legumes such as lentils, beans and peas) will ensure you get sufficient fibre, which acts as food for your gut microbes. It is best to increase the amount of fibre you eat gradually to allow your digestive system to adapt to the change. Often referred to as prebiotics, plant fibre is a source of food for the microbes and helps to support a healthy digestive system, which in turn influences so many aspects of health that scientists are just starting to understand. A healthy gut microbiome doesn't only protect you from gut problems, but it has also been linked to immunity, brain health, metabolic health and more. Eating foods that contain live microbes, such as natural yoghurt, kimchi, sauerkraut and kefir, may help the gut microbiome, and many nutritionists recommend adding these fermented foods to the diet. The microbes these foods contain are referred to as probiotics and they are also available in supplement form. Whether they can get from your mouth to the right part of your digestive system (the large intestine) is a matter for debate and you will see some products advertised with the claim 'gets to the gut alive'. This is currently an area of nutritional science interest so I am sure you will hear more and more about it in the future.

Protein

Another factor to consider is to ensure you get enough protein-rich foods. There are some chemicals our bodies can't make, including protein building blocks known as 'essential amino acids'. These are amino acids that we must eat because our bodies can't manufacture them. Meat proteins usually have all of these essential amino acids, so it is easy to get them all if you are a meat or fish eater. We can get all of the essential amino acids from plants, but you need to combine different plants to ensure you get all of them. This means vegans and vegetarians need to be a bit more careful about getting enough protein and the Vegan Society[2] provides information to help. So have a think about the sources of protein in each of your meals. You don't need to eat very high quantities or take a supplement, as a balanced diet will usually provide sufficient protein. There are, however, debates in the nutrition world about how much protein we need, so if you are concerned about whether you are getting enough protein in your diet, do find out the most up-to-date research from a reliable source.

Older people are recommended to increase their protein intake as they start to lose muscle as they age. It is very important to keep strong muscles through eating sufficient protein and doing strength training. This is to prevent weakness affecting how we live our lives (see *5:B Stay active*). You want to be able to carry shopping, move about easily, enjoy your hobbies and manage in your own home. You may also want to be able to put your suitcase into the overhead locker of a plane! This is one of my personal goals for old age, so that I can travel independently until I am in my 90s or older. It may seem like an unrealistic dream, but I certainly hope it is one I can fulfil.

Higher amounts of protein are also recommended for people who are doing a lot of strength training and focusing on building muscle. Be aware that excess protein is used for energy or stored as fat, so it is best not to take protein shakes or supplements unless you are advised to do so for a specific reason by a dietician.

Healthy fats

You also need to ensure you are getting healthy fats. There are some 'essential' fatty acids. These are components of fats that we can't manufacture in the body and that we need to get from our diet. There are lots of good fats, such as those found in oily fish, nuts and seeds, and also in minimally processed oils such as extra virgin olive oil and cold pressed oils. Seed oils, however, are an area where there is disagreement about whether they are harmful to health or not.[3,4] I avoid them where possible as I try to follow the principle of minimal processing, and these oils are highly processed – 'typically created through synthetic chemical extraction methods that sometimes include additional processing like bleaching and deodorising'.[5] Examples include vegetable, sunflower, and rapeseed (canola) oils. Contrary to what you may have heard, extra-virgin olive oil is fine for cooking as well as for using cold and is associated with many health benefits, so if you can afford it, this is the best oil for health.

There is still some disagreement over whether saturated fat is linked to heart disease, with evidence being produced both for and against,[6,7] so maybe saturated fat, for now, should be eaten in moderation. Certainly there are a number of experts who blame refined carbohydrates, such as sugars and starchy foods,[8] for the high levels of heart disease in our modern populations, rather than saturated fat. You will find all of the arguments online if you care to look. I favour a moderate amount of saturated fat from minimally processed sources, such as simple cuts of meat, full fat yoghurt and good cheeses. Definitely none of your overly processed cheese strings! There seems to be no doubt that trans fats, and hydrogenated fats, (made by using hydrogen to turn liquid oils into solid fats) are bad for us and should be avoided.

Meat
The use of nitrates and nitrites in the curing of processed meats, such as sausages, bacon, ham and salami, have been linked to an increased risk of colon cancer,[9] so eat these less frequently. Red meat generally should not be eaten too often

as, again, it is linked with an increased risk of colon cancer. NHS guidelines[10] suggest 70g a day as the maximum, so having some red-meat-free days is a good idea (70g of bacon is about 1.5 rashers, so not a huge amount). There are no guidelines for white meat such as chicken.

The production of red meat has a high carbon footprint so reducing the amount you eat is good for your health and good for the planet too. Red meat does have valuable nutrients such as complete protein, iron, vitamin B12 and others so moderation is probably the best advice. Eating locally reared meat is also better for you and the planet, so a small amount of high-quality meat from your butcher or farm shop can be a part of a healthy meal.

Salt

There are guidelines about the maximum amount of salt that should be in our diets. The recommended maximum per day is 6g or about a teaspoon.[11] I thought this was one area that all the experts agreed on – that salt can cause issues such as high blood pressure and kidney problems[12] – and then I heard Professor Tim Spector saying on a podcast[13] that salt was not an issue after all. When I started looking into the literature, I found that there were studies showing no conclusive evidence that salt increased the risk of heart disease,[14] but others saying the opposite,[15] so it is hard to know what to believe. If you are eating unprocessed food, and you cook most of your meals yourself, you are unlikely to have a high intake of salt unless you add it into your cooking or at the table. I am shocked at some TV chefs who seem to throw handfuls of salt into their cooking. So, cook for yourself and this is something you can easily control. Now pass me a packet of salted nuts – with all this talk of food I am feeling rather peckish!

Carbohydrates

Another area of controversy in the diet world concerns carbohydrate-rich foods. These include foods high in sugar or starch. Starch gets broken down in the body into sugars. There are no essential carbohydrates, as our body can manufacture the ones we need from proteins and fats, and this knowledge has led to the argument that we don't need to eat many carb-rich foods. As a result, low-carb diets have become very popular. So should we eat carbs, such as wheat-based products like bread and pasta or natural carb-heavy foods like potatoes and rice? Firstly it is our body's preferred energy source, so you could argue our body needs carbs for energy. One helpful question to ask is how you feel when you eat them. If you have no problem with them, that is great. Eat them in moderation. I find if I have a lunch that is high in carbohydrates, such as a sandwich, I tend to feel quite tired in the afternoon. Some people seem to fare better with lower carb levels, and this is certainly advocated by some clinicians in the treatment of Type 2 diabetes.[16]

Before we demonise carbs altogether, there are some communities that eat high levels of carbohydrates and live long, healthy lives. Dan Buettner has studied five communities around the world that have a high proportion of centenarians. He calls these areas 'Blue Zones'[17] and he discovered that they thrive on high-carb diets. Their carbs are mainly whole grains, greens and beans rather than refined carbs and sugar. So if you do like carb-rich foods, try to eat wholegrain rather than white flour products, and reduce the amount of refined sugar in your diet. We do know that excess sugar consumption is one of the factors that can lead to obesity, which increases the risk of developing Type 2 diabetes[18] and other conditions,[19] so have sweet stuff sparingly. If you do want a sweet treat, try to get it from whole fruit rather than sweets and biscuits. If you love cake, then try to make your own, and bear in mind there are now so many recipes available for healthier sweet treat options. One of my favourite sweet treats is a square of dark chocolate, spread with pure peanut or almond butter (no additives) and topped with a few raisins.

When you consider your nutrition, it is important to ask yourself some questions. Is my way of eating working for me? Am I healthy, lean and energetic? Is my immune system strong? Is my digestion regular and calm? If not, then focus on making the majority of your food minimally processed and seek out a nutritionist or dietician if you feel you need help to improve your diet.

Eat thoughtfully

The next elements of healthy eating I want to consider are not about types of food but about ways of eating. The first one is to eat thoughtfully. How often do we just eat mindlessly? You have a packet of crisps or some chocolate and the first few mouthfuls are delicious, but I know for me that if I actually analyse what the tenth mouthful tastes like, it usually does not taste nearly so good. When we eat mindlessly we are more likely to overeat.[20]

Fasting

You may also have seen increasing coverage in the health news about types of fasting. Time restricted eating (TRE) is growing in popularity and is the subject of much research. This involves only eating in a restricted time window, maybe 8 or 10 hours, with a maximum of 12. So you might want to give this a try as it is thought to have a range of health benefits, such as cell and immune system repair and regulation of blood sugar.[21] You can find lots of articles on the benefits of fasting on the internet, but don't forget to look for the downsides too before deciding if it might be worth trying. TRE is something I have adopted. I found it quite difficult at first but after a few weeks I found it very easy. Because I like to have dinner after work in the evening, I now don't eat breakfast but I have lunch about 12 or 1pm, and this has made maintaining my weight easy, plus I feel I have more energy in the morning. Before I started TRE I would often get really hungry mid-morning and mid-afternoon, despite eating breakfast and lunch, and I really felt like I could not function until I had a snack, but that has gone away now. No more getting hangry mid-afternoon! It would be preferable to have my eating window earlier in the day as this regime has shown greater health benefits, but for me that does not work as I like to eat my main meal in the evening.

An easier way to gain some of the benefits of TRE is to restrict food intake to 12 hours a day, maybe stopping eating at 7.30pm and not having breakfast until 7.30am. Giving our digestive systems some time to rest and repair seems to be a good idea.[22] Breakfast has long been hailed as the most important meal of the day, but I like to consider that concept in the light of evolution. Our ancestors did not have cupboards and fridges full of food available when they woke up. I am sure they would have had to go and get food for their family before having something to eat, so we are perfectly capable of functioning for some time before needing to eat. In fact, we get a natural increase in glucose in the blood in the morning, which provides some energy.[23] I think the key message is to do what is right for you, and maybe try out some different options and see how they make you feel. We are all different.

Another fasting regime you may have heard about is the 5:2 diet, where on two days a week calories are kept very low – 600 for men and 500 for women. Again, good health benefits have been associated with this regime. You might have seen Michael Mosley's book[24] explaining the science behind it. I have given it a try but I found the low calorie days very difficult and could not maintain this pattern of eating but I know people who have eaten that way for years. Again, play around and see what works for you. The important thing with these fasting regimes is to make sure you eat a nutritious diet. Also, it is important to consider that these restricted regimes may not be suitable for people with any health issues or issues around eating disorders, women at certain stages of the menstrual cycle, menopausal women and people doing high levels of exercise. Do read more about fasting and potential side effects and problems before giving any of the regimes a try. See resources for books on fasting.

Drinking

I also want us to consider what we drink. I think you know I'm going to say don't have ultra-processed drinks such as fizzy drinks with sugars or sweeteners. There are lots of differing thoughts on whether sweeteners are bad for you, but personally I avoid them as they are far too processed for me. The World Health Organisation has recently added aspartame to their list of potential carcinogens[25] and there is some evidence that they may interfere adversely with the gut microbiome.[26] They can also help to maintain a sweet tooth, which can mean we are more likely to eat sugary food. I also think we need to be cautious about drinking lots of calories. I don't generally like to focus on calories, because we can't tell how the calories listed on a packet relate to the energy our body actually gets to use. But many of the sweetened coffee drinks, hot chocolates, juices and smoothies from high street coffee shops contain lots of energy (calories), which can add up over the course of a week. If you are struggling to maintain a healthy weight it is worth having a think about whether you are having high calorie drinks, and then try to swap them for water, plain tea or coffee.

On the subject of drinking, we need to stay well hydrated for our bodies to work properly; after all we are about 60% water. But we also need to be aware that we can overhydrate, which is not good for us either. More fluid than the body can cope with leads to a sodium imbalance, which can be very harmful and ultimately fatal[27] – and this has happened during marathon running.[28] UK guidelines recommend drinking 6–8 mugs a day, and this includes the water in tea, coffee and food, but again you will find different opinions regarding hydration, with some experts claiming that the focus on hydration is just a marketing ploy by drinks companies[29]. But having drinks throughout the day is certainly important, and the best thing is to drink regularly and listen to your thirst signals. They are there to tell us we need to drink more water. You will need more if it is hot, or you are exercising. Older adults may not recognise they are thirsty, so they may need prompting to ensure they drink enough.

Alcohol

What about alcohol? If you do drink alcohol, stick to the guidelines of a maximum of 14 units per week with a number of alcohol-free days.[30] I enjoy a glass or two of wine and the way I keep track of how much I drink at home is to pour a set amount of wine into a mini-carafe and stick to that. Large measures served at home can be difficult to monitor, so this is my way of keeping track. It works really well for me. There are also many alcohol-free beers, fizz and spirit substitutes that are well worth trying out, but I have yet to find a good alcohol-free red or white wine substitute. And if you do think you have an alcohol problem, please seek help. There is a lot of help available from various organisations, both local and national, as well as a number of groups on social media that provide motivation and support to cut down or give up alcohol.[31]

Other issues

Another thing to consider with trying to eat healthily is that we often eat for reasons other than hunger – whether it is because of boredom or habit, at social gatherings or for comfort. There are certainly no simple solutions to these particular food issues, and I am not covering them here as it is not something I have any training or expertise in, so if you do have issues around emotional eating or an eating disorder, please try and seek some help from a therapist or your GP.

There is so much written about diet and healthy eating, much of it conflicting, so I am only touching the surface here, but I really believe it does not have to be that complicated. Eat slowly and thoughtfully, choose unprocessed foods, or process food yourself (by that I mean cook), eat lots of vegetables and try to have a wide variety. Try not to snack, but if you must snack, eat whole foods such as a piece of fruit or a few unsalted nuts. If you stick to this most of the time, you can't go far wrong. We all have occasions when we want to eat less-healthy food, so go ahead and have the cake, the chocolate, the burger, etc. guilt free. If they are only minor parts of your diet, you won't need to worry. I also realise that for so many people it is hard to find the time to cook, or they don't have suitable cooking facilities, or the shops nearby mostly sell ultra-processed foods. Under these circumstances it is much harder to eat healthily, but even small changes, when options allow, can help to improve your health. Keep on doing your best.

Supplements

Finally, if you are eating a well-balanced, varied, whole food diet you shouldn't need any extra vitamins or minerals, with the exception of vitamin D in the winter (10 micrograms per day is recommended by the UK government),[32] and vitamin

B12 for vegans.[33] However, there is some evidence that our food contains fewer vitamins and minerals than in the past,[34] due to the intensive nature of farming, so a multivitamin and mineral supplement might be an insurance policy. Do take time to read more about them if you decide to go down the route of taking supplements, as they can also cause harm, and so many of them are not tested for safety. There are many reports that vitamin and mineral supplements just make expensive urine, but recently a few studies are starting to point in the direction of some benefits for multivitamins, so this is one area I am watching with interest. In particular, one study suggested that a daily multivitamin may reduce cognitive decline.[35]

Before we go on to the next milestone, I want you to spend a few minutes considering a typical day's food and whether there are easy ways to reduce how much ultra-processed food you eat. I have given a few examples below.

Breakfast
Basic: Instant porridge with golden syrup
Better: Oats with dried fruit
Even better: Jumbo organic oats with full fat Greek yoghurt, fresh fruit, nuts and seeds

Lunch
Basic: White bread ham sandwich, crisps, fizzy drink
Better: Wholegrain bread tuna salad sandwich, apple, tea or water
Even better: Salmon and bean salad (with lots of vegetables), extra virgin olive oil dressing, fruit salad, tea or water

Dinner (*meat*)

Basic: Cheeseburger in white roll, chips from a take-away, fizzy drink

Better: Home-cooked burger, burger bun, cheese slice, oven chips, orange juice

Even better: Home-made burger, Cheddar cheese, mixed salad, potato wedges, water

Dinner (*fish*)

Basic: Fish and chips from a take-away, fizzy drink

Better: Home cooked fish, oven chips, orange juice

Even better: Salmon cooked on a bed of mixed vegetables (onion, peppers, mushrooms, courgette, leeks), new potatoes, water

Dinner (*vegetarian/vegan*)

Basic: Vegan burger in a white roll, chips from a take-away, fizzy drink

Better: Oven cooked vegan burger, burger bun, tomato ketchup, oven chips, orange juice

Even better: Homemade vegan burger made from beans, lentils and vegetables, salad, sweet potato wedges, water

Snack

Basic: Two chocolate digestive biscuits

Better: One chocolate digestive biscuit and half an apple

Even better: A square of 70% dark chocolate, half an apple, a few unsalted mixed nuts

Hopefully I have encouraged you to think about whether you need to eat fewer ultra-processed foods and drinks and have given you some ideas for small changes that can make a big difference. Remember that nutritional advice is always changing, but by focusing on real, whole food you can't go far wrong.

And while this path is called look after my body, by taking care of what you eat you will also be benefitting your mind, as what we eat affects not only our physical health but, importantly, our mental health too. The food you eat affects your mood as well as your energy levels and waistline. For detailed information on the effects of food on the brain and mental health, have a read of Felice Jacka's book *Brain Changer* or Christopher Palmer's *Brain Energy*.

5:B – Stay active

Please take care if starting any new exercise regime and check with your doctor or physiotherapist first. Make sure that you build up very gradually and have rest days for recovery.

I am sure you will have seen some of the scary headlines, such as 'sitting is the new smoking', and I must admit I take all of these simplistic storylines with a pinch of salt (no more than 6g of course!). But there is no denying that staying active is vitally important if we want to keep healthy. When I trained as an exercise teacher for older adults[36] we focused on four key areas of activity – flexibility, aerobic fitness, balance and strength. Easily remembered as FABS! So let us look at each of these in a bit more detail.

As I mentioned above do be careful when starting any new exercise regime and check with your doctor if you are in any doubt about whether an exercise is suitable for you. We are all different with varying bodies and health conditions so please be cautious. Be aware that over-exercising is not good for you either[37] but, having said that, it is being inactive that is causing many health problems, so let's get started!

Flexibility

What do you do to keep flexible? Perhaps you go to a yoga or Pilates class, do some stretches at home, or maybe you never think about it until one day you try to bend down to tie up your shoelace and you feel awkward, stiff and old. Hopefully that is not how you feel, but many people do feel that way – and from a surprisingly young age. For women the perimenopause years can signal the start of joint and muscle pain due to changing hormone levels. So, whilst older age inevitably comes with some changes to our bodies, it is important to keep flexible so that you can have an active older age, one where you can continue to live the life you want, and one that has fewer aches and pains.

Fortunately, there are many resources that are easily available to help us with maintaining flexibility. You may have access to a yoga or Pilates class near where you live, and these are great ways of supporting you to be flexible and supple. I am in awe of the over-80s who attend the yoga and Pilates classes I attend, and that they can perform all of the exercises better than I can. They are a real inspiration to me and remove any doubts from my mind that you can have a strong, flexible body into old age. If you can't get to a class there are free videos on YouTube, and the NHS website has a variety of exercises that you can follow. Try to get into the habit of starting each day with a short exercise routine. My morning routine has been developed from attending Pilates and yoga classes, plus exercises my physiotherapist gave me to do when I had a sore back, or sore neck, over the years. It takes no more than 10 or 15 minutes, but it makes such a difference to how I feel. I often speak to clients who are suffering from a sore back, and they have had many visits to the physio at considerable expense, but when their initial pain has subsided they forget all about the exercises the physio gave them and return to 'normal'. Unfortunately, 'normal' is not thinking about looking after their back, until the next painful episode. If they incorporated the exercises into a daily routine, they would be less likely to hurt their back again. If they do, they are likely to recover more quickly. So think of any physio visits you have as lessons about the exercises you need to do every day, not as a few sessions of treatment that are to be forgotten. The same applies to sore knees, neck, feet, etc. Most days I do the exercises my podiatrist gave me for an Achilles problem, and I have had no reoccurrence of the pain since. (I will probably have just jinxed myself and will be hobbling about next week!) For the flexibility of all your muscles and joints, spend a bit of time working out what is right for you and make sure it is part of your everyday life.

Another important area to consider is the effect of your working environment. As much as possible, make sure your working conditions don't cause you problems with your posture. If you sit down all day, make sure you get up regularly to move about and stretch. Can you set a timer so that you get up at least every hour, if not every half hour? Do you remember the Pomodoro technique from *2:C Manage my time*?

Another option is to have a sit-to-stand desk. You can buy an expensive one that goes up and down at the touch of a button or a manual one with a crank handle. The latter is the type I have, and I consider the manual part as an extra activity for my arm muscles. I just paused my typing to crank up my desk as I realised that I had not stood up at my desk today and it is 2pm. I usually have some time standing in the morning and in the afternoon, but it does tend to depend on what I am doing. I usually sit down for meetings and stand for working at my computer.

Having a soft surface to stand on is recommended, so you may need to buy a mat if you have a hard floor rather than a carpet. Make sure that you set up your desk correctly, so do look for some guidance on the internet where you will find information about the suggested height of the desk and position of your computer, so that you avoid causing yourself any injuries which would rather defeat the purpose. Make sure any advice you follow from the internet is from a reputable source such as a physiotherapy organisation. If you are unsure if a sit-to-stand desk is right for you, discuss it with a physiotherapist, or the member of staff at your work who is responsible for safe ergonomics. And start slowly with short periods of time standing so that you get used to it gradually. Standing all day is not great for you either,[38] so variety is the thing to aim for.

If your job involves lots of time spent in the car, again take regular breaks to stretch out your muscles, and make sure your seat is in the best position for your back and neck. Many working days are lost due to back pain, so ensuring you are giving your muscles and joints the priority they need can save you a lot of pain and inconvenience in the long run.

Aerobic fitness

The Department of Health[39] recommends adults get at least 150 minutes of moderate aerobic activity, such as cycling or brisk walking, every week, or 75 minutes of vigorous exercise such as running. (You may have heard the advice to get at least 30 minutes of exercise on five days a week, and that equates to the 150 minutes from the guidelines.) Many people find that having a step count monitor is motivating. I certainly find that sitting all morning and having done only about 1,000 steps is a wake-up call to get moving. The figure of 10,000 steps is a fairly arbitrary number, and I occasionally read of studies[40] that suggest a different target to aim for, but the important thing is to stay active. You will also have heard all of the usual advice such as using the stairs rather than the lift, parking further from the shops or getting off the bus a stop early. This is to encourage you to add in lots of little bursts of activity throughout the day. They really do add up. Dr Rangan Chatterjee, in his book *Feel Better in 5*, calls these shorts bursts of activity 'health snacks', so adding in lots of health snacks during the day is a great way to improve your overall physical health.

High intensity interval training (HIIT) has received a lot of publicity in recent years as a good way of improving fitness.

One scientifically validated routine[41] is the seven-minute HIIT routine and there are a number of apps which guide you through this. I thought, 'Seven minutes – how hard can it be?' but it is actually quite hard. Well, it was for me! You get lots of benefit in a short time, which is great for busy people, but certainly not an easy option for those who have not exercised for a while. If you do give it a try, start off gently and build up gradually to the full routine.

Running has also become increasingly popular in recent times, thanks largely to Parkrun, which is a free weekly timed 5K event on Saturday mornings. Have a look for your local Parkrun. You can walk, jog or run and it is a great way to start the weekend. The NHS also has a Couch to 5K programme that can help you get started, and there are local running groups you can join. I started running about nine years ago and love my local Parkrun. A big thank you to my local St Andrews Parkrun directors and other volunteers who are there whatever the weather. I often do run/walk/run, which is known as 'Jeffing' after Jeff Galloway, who pioneered this method. It's much easier than constant running and gentler on the body, so have a look at that option if you think running is not for you. I run for 60 seconds and walk for 30 seconds and I really love that. I intend to keep Jeffing forever rather than return to continuous running, as it is definitely easier on the body. I don't tend to get injured with Jeffing and it is more sociable as you can easily chat away to your running buddies whilst still raising your heartrate and getting the aerobic benefits. A big shout out here to my local running group the Anster Allsorts who have kept me motivated to keep running, as without my running friends I am sure I would have given up by now.

There are so many different forms of aerobic exercise, from brisk walking to dancing to cycling and all of the team sports. The most important thing is to find something you enjoy and can continue over the long term. Maybe you like walking or cycling or playing tennis, or maybe you love your local dance class or like to go swimming. The key thing is to find something you can sustain and then build that into your daily life. Also be aware that it is important to ensure that you do some weight-bearing exercise to guard against the development of osteoporosis.

So have a think about what you currently do for your aerobic health and ask yourself if you are doing enough to maintain good aerobic fitness. If you are honest with yourself, you will know if you can easily run for the bus, walk up a hill or keep up with friends who walk briskly. Remember, if you think you need to do more than you do at the moment, start small and gradually increase, or you are likely to get demotivated or, even worse, injured. As in most things, you can overdo exercise, so stick to the NHS guidelines and build up gradually and you won't go far wrong. Remember to build in recovery time, which is especially important as you get older. If you are unsure about what you should do, then check with your doctor or a physiotherapist.

Balance

Let's look at the third area of FABS – balance. Here is a test you can try at home. **Please be careful and only try this if you can do so safely.**

Stand on one leg and time how long you can stand for. If you manage over a minute you can stop. Then try the other leg. Now repeat the test but this time with your eyes closed. Take care you don't fall and injure yourself – you have been warned!

So how did you get on? Our ability to balance declines as we get older. A study in the Journal of Geriatric Physical Therapy[42] looked at the ability to balance at different ages and the data is shown in the table below.

If you struggled balancing with your eyes open or closed, then this is something to add into your daily routine. Balance is very important for preventing falls when we are older, so it is best to work on it now to prevent problems in the future. You can get balance boards to incorporate into a home routine, but you don't need to get that fancy, as a daily balance practice added to the end of your morning exercises will certainly help. I balance on each leg for 30 seconds with my eyes closed. I often have to touch my foot down when I lose my balance, but I just start again until I have done a total of 30 seconds. Some days are better than others!

Age	Average time eyes open (seconds)	Average time eyes closed (seconds)
18–39	43	9
40–49	40	7
50–59	37	5
60–69	27	3
70–79	15	2
80–99	6	1

Yoga and Pilates are also great for improving balance. I am sure you have seen pictures of people in a tree posture at yoga, balancing on one leg. There are lots of other balance postures in yoga too, some of them surprisingly difficult. You might find that adding in a balance while you are brushing your teeth could help make it part of your routine. But be careful and don't take any risks. Falls are a major cause of loss of independence and even death.[43]

Strength
The fourth element of FABS is strength. We start to lose muscle strength in our 30s,[44] so it is important to try and maintain our strength by doing some simple weight-bearing exercises such as squats, lunges, planks and push-ups. All of these exercises are part of the seven-minute HIIT routine mentioned previously, and you will also find examples of strength exercises on the internet. Just make sure you pick a reputable resource such as the NHS Fitness Studio in the UK.[45]

I do a few arm strengthening exercises using dumbbells every morning, but you don't need to use any equipment as you can just use your own bodyweight to improve your strength, or you can use items around the house like food tins and bottles of water. One of the benefits of using dumbbells is that you can see the progression as you gradually increase the weight you can lift. Be careful that you don't overdo it. Start with a light weight and increase as your muscles get stronger. If you are in any doubt, speak to a physiotherapist or gym instructor. I really advise that you listen to your body. I know of a few people who have ended up badly injured from attending a gym where they were encouraged to lift weights that were too heavy for them. There is no benefit in starting off with heavy weights and then having to give up due to injury. My mantra is this: what can I keep doing consistently into old age? This still incorporates getting stronger and fitter over time, but not getting into a cycle of exercise followed by injury. I am lifting stronger weights than when I started, and I hope to always be strong enough to lift that 10kg suitcase into the overhead luggage compartment on a plane! Having real-life, practical goals for your fitness regime can really help to keep you motivated.

Grip strength

As we get older we also lose grip strength in our hands and end up struggling to open jars and carry heavy bags. Grip strength is also used as an indicator of overall health in older adults. You can measure your grip strength with a dynamometer, and this is something I take along to my workshops so participants can measure their strength. You can buy grip strengtheners; I use mine at the end of my morning routine and my grip strength has increased so that I now register as 'strong' on the dynamometer. That makes me happy! Keeping a stress ball on your desk, so you can give it a squeeze every now and again, can also be a good way of exercising your fingers.

Pelvic floor

It is also important to keep your pelvic floor muscles strong. Performing regular exercises can help to guard against incontinence in later life and improve your sex life. Pelvic floor exercises are often focused on women, but they are very important for men too. Men – keep reading! There are two types of muscles to focus on: fast twitch and slow twitch. For the slow twitch muscles, you can sit or stand, then draw up the back passage as if to stop passing wind, then bring this sensation around to the front passage as if trying to stop passing urine. Hold for 10 seconds, then release slowly. Rest for three or four seconds, then repeat, building up to 10 repetitions. For fast twitch, draw up the pelvic floor muscles as fast as possible, hold for a second, then release and repeat 10 times. Men may find it helpful to imagine pulling up their trouser zip. If you are having problems with your pelvic floor muscles, do seek help from a specialist physiotherapist or your GP.

So that is our quick look at staying physically active. Flexibility, aerobic fitness, balance and strength. Spend a few more minutes having a think about what you do now and if there is anything you need to add into your life. If you start to think, 'I will start that next month,' then whatever you are planning to do is just too ambitious. It needs to be something you can start in the next day or two and something that does not feel like a big change in your life. It also needs to be something that you can continue to do for the rest of your life (or a moderated version of it), otherwise I guarantee that you will give up. Start small and be consistent – that is the most important thing. And don't forget that if you have any health concerns at all you should speak to your doctor or physio before you begin any new exercise regime.

5:C – Sleep well

Sleep has been the subject of many health articles lately as more and more research is helping us to understand what goes on overnight while we sleep. So how long should you aim to sleep for? Matthew Walker, in his best-selling book *Why We Sleep*, recommends having an eight-hour 'sleep opportunity'. All that means is having time in bed trying to sleep (not reading or on your phone). So have a think about how long you are lying down in bed with the lights off and work out how long your sleep opportunity is on a normal night. I usually go to bed about 10.30/11pm and the alarm goes off at 6.30am, so that gives me the recommended sleep opportunity if I am at the earlier end of my bedtime. I probably get about seven-and-a-half hours of sleep out of that eight-hour sleep opportunity. We are all different, and the eight hours is a guide, with different people needing different amounts of sleep.[46] The important thing is to know how well you are functioning during the day and whether you need to give your sleep a greater priority.

If you don't have any trouble sleeping, meaning you are out like a light as soon as your head hits the pillow, and you wake naturally a few minutes before the alarm, you can skip this section and head straight over to Path 6 – and consider yourself very lucky! This section really won't be of much interest and may make you overthink your sleep, so take my advice and move on. For those of you who class yourself as someone who does not sleep well, bear with me and we will look at some tips for helping to improve your sleep.

Why should we focus on getting a good night's sleep? Poor sleep quality is linked to an increased risk of a number of health issues such as heart conditions and even dementia.[47,48] If you are not a great sleeper it does not mean you will suffer from these diseases, but it does mean you should make an effort to improve your chances of a good sleep. I recently read an obituary of a 94-year-old who was a 'lifelong insomniac' – something so well known about her that the writer thought to mention it in her obituary, but she still lived to a very old age! So if you aren't a great sleeper, do your best to follow the guidance for improving sleep, but try not to worry. When people are analysed in sleep labs they often get much more sleep than they realise,[49] so relax, don't worry and just do your best. A note of caution, however: if a lack of sleep is making your life dangerous, such as having microsleeps when driving, then do speak to your GP urgently to identify underlying causes such as sleep apnoea.

Now before you go any further, answer the questions below to assess how well you sleep and to see whether you need to make some changes to help with your sleep. Answer each question using the following scoring, then work out the total out of 10.

Scoring

Rarely or never = 0   Sometimes = 1   Always = 2

1. Do you wake up feeling refreshed*?
2. Do you stay awake all day without dozing?
3. Do you wake at roughly the same time each day without an alarm (within 30 minutes).
4. Do you fall asleep within 30 minutes?
5. Do you get back to sleep easily if you wake in the night?

*After the initial morning grogginess or sleep inertia has worn off – usually within 20–30 minutes.[50]

Obviously the lower the score, the more important it is to try to improve your chances of a good night's sleep. But remember that sleep is not an active process that you can control, like going out for a walk; all you can do is give yourself the best chance and then relax and try not to worry about it.

So what happens overnight when we are in the land of nod? Sleep strengthens the immune system, boosts your metabolism and balances your hormones. Sleep also removes waste products from the brain and helps to store memories. It is important for regulating your emotions. I am certainly less patient when I am tired, so you may well recognise that you are a bit more easily angered or irritated after a bad night's sleep. Hunger hormones are also disrupted by poor sleep. Do you ever feel hungrier in the morning if you are tired? I know that I do. There are many processes that happen in the body and brain when we sleep, so if you want to know more about this, then take a look at one of the books I list in the resources section.

What can help us sleep? We will look at tips for two main types of sleep disturbances. Firstly there are people who have difficulty getting off to sleep, and secondly there are those who can get off to sleep but wake in the night and struggle to get back to sleep. The latter disturbance is called difficulty with 'sleep maintenance'. Some people of course have both. For each tip below, have a think about whether this is something you do already or something you might try.

Get sunlight in the morning

A good night's sleep starts in the morning with getting sunlight first thing. Could you walk part of your journey to work, or sit and have a coffee outside, wrapped up warm? Getting light early in the day resets your body clock, so try to avoid wearing sunglasses in the morning.

Limit screens in the evening

I am sure you will have heard all of the warnings about avoiding screens at night, as the blue light is thought to affect the sleep process.[51] I have seen some research that disputes this,[52] but ask yourself if screen use could be affecting your sleep. Try a week with turning your phone off an hour or two before bed and don't take it into the bedroom. Then analyse how that worked for you. Because we are all so different, it is often worth evaluating health advice by asking yourself if it is working for you. Sometimes, however, we can't see the impact of our behaviour until many years down the line, so we might need to take the experts' advice. Smoking is a perfect example as it can take years before the effects are felt, so it's best to trust the experts on that. But I often say to my coaching clients to 'be your own detective'. What works for you might not work for someone else – listen to your body and your mind!

Avoid caffeine

Avoiding caffeine from lunchtime is another good piece of advice. Caffeine takes about six hours to reduce by half in your body, so if you are really sensitive to caffeine you might have to avoid it or switch to decaffeinated all day, but experiment and see what works for you. Some people are not at all sensitive to caffeine and others are very sensitive. Again, know what works for you. My husband can drink a double espresso half an hour before bedtime and not notice any impact on his sleep, whereas I would be awake half the night after a single shot. Most annoying!

Avoid alcohol

You will probably know that alcohol interferes with sleep. It can send you off to sleep but then wake you in the night, and it doesn't induce a natural sleep. So having alcohol-free days, not drinking too much and avoiding alcohol close to bedtime is important for a restful night's sleep.

Look after your body

The other topics we have covered in Path 5 – that is eating healthily and exercising – are also important for good sleep, but try not to do either of these too late in the evening. Late exercise can make it harder to relax and cool down sufficiently to go off to sleep. Eating late can also disrupt the process of getting to sleep, so try to finish eating 2–3 hours before bedtime.

Healthy lifestyle

It may be obvious, but it is worth stating that a healthy lifestyle will also benefit your sleep. Keeping to a healthy weight can help to reduce the likelihood of snoring or sleep apnoea interfering with your sleep. Whilst not everyone who snores or who has sleep apnoea is overweight, the likelihood of both of these conditions is greater in people who are overweight.

Smoking is another lifestyle factor that affects sleep. Smoking reduces the depth and length of sleep and nicotine cravings can wake smokers up during the night. There is so much help available to quit smoking, so do speak to your pharmacist if you smoke and would like to quit.

Sleep schedule

Try to establish a regular sleep routine: going to bed and getting up at the same time every day. Yes, even weekends! Maintaining a regular sleep and wake time all week is one of the best ways of improving sleep. Ideally go to bed early enough so that you wake just before the alarm. This will help to set your circadian rhythm (biological clock) and make it easier to go to sleep at night.

Pre-bedtime routine

Having a calming pre-bedtime routine can be very helpful. Try not to engage in any activity that can get you 'worked up'. Don't read your work emails, watch something distressing or too exciting on the TV, or start discussing emotional topics with your loved ones. Instead aim for a calming wind-down process about an hour before bed. Maybe do some meditation, read a good book or have a bath with Epsom salts and lavender oil. Or maybe have a shower followed by a slow, gentle yoga routine. Or maybe spend some time writing down a few things you are grateful for in your life, or a few things that have gone well that day. Then go off to sleep thinking positive thoughts.

Sleepy bedroom

Another tip is to make your bedroom a peaceful haven. Make sure your mattress and pillows are comfortable and the room is cool and dark. Temperature is important, as too hot a sleeping environment is not conducive to dropping off to sleep. Don't watch TV or use electronics in the bedroom if possible. It is best to make it purely a place for sleep and romance, (and a morning cup of tea). ☺ This is so you associate the bedroom with a place of relaxation rather than alertness. This can of course be difficult as some people need to work or study in their bedroom, but where possible confine activities that tend to keep you awake to another room. You may need some electronics, such as your phone, if you are using them to play sleep-inducing, soothing music or maybe an audio bedtime story. There are some apps that have special stories to help you go off to sleep. I occasionally use 'sleep stories' on the Headspace app if I have trouble sleeping. There are lots of different stories with different narrators; you just need to find the most soporific one. If you find that having your phone in the bedroom to play sleep stories means you end up scrolling through social media at four in the morning, then it is best to completely ban the phone from the bedroom at night. Maybe you can find an old-fashioned way to play a relaxing story or music, such as a CD player. That might be too much of a challenge! It is also really important to have children's and teenagers' bedrooms as tech-free zones at night, as sleep is so essential for the developing mind and body. I know that is not an easy rule to impose, but sometimes parents need to be strong when they know it is in the best interests of their child.

Keep cool

Your core body temperature needs to drop to send you off to sleep. A hot bath or shower, about 90 minutes before bedtime, helps to reduce your temperature and makes you feel sleepy. It seems counter-intuitive, but the hot bath sends more blood from your core to the surface of the skin, and this results in the body cooling down. I certainly know I look rather pink after a bath; the result of that increased blood flow to my skin.

Once you are in bed, having cool, cotton bed linen and thin cotton nightclothes can help too. You can also buy cooling mats and pillows for your bed, and I know many people who love these, especially women going through the menopause. When I became perimenopausal, one thing that I really noticed was the change in how hot I felt at night. I went from someone who needed a thick duvet, even in the summer, to someone who didn't need any cover, even in the winter. Quite a change! I would often moan that my thermostat was broken. Making changes to what I wore in bed and adding a sheet under a light duvet meant I had a number of different thermal layers to choose from in the night. So do experiment if this sounds familiar. It really can help.

If you are very hot due to being in a hot country or due to menopausal symptoms, wet a pillowcase or a thin towel and use that as a blanket, or spray a top sheet with water. This has saved me on many a holiday without air conditioning. It might sound weird, but it is really very effective. Again, it is all about the body being cool enough to allow you to drop off to sleep.

Dark and quiet bedroom

It is important to have a dark and quiet place to sleep, but that is not always easy to control. Using an eye mask and ear plugs can be very helpful, especially when you are travelling. I am a very light sleeper, so I never travel without my mask and ear plugs (I like soft silicone ones). Ear plugs can be helpful if your partner snores!

Distract your mind

Many people find reading a book or listening to an audio book or the radio can help them fall asleep as it distracts the mind from other thoughts that might keep them awake. Just make sure to set a timer so that it turns off automatically.

Meditation and relaxation

If you have trouble getting off to sleep or you wake up and can't get back to sleep, meditation can help. Now for this to really work you need to get into the habit of regular meditation. The sessions don't have to be long, but like any new skill it needs to be practised. Again, there are apps to help, and we will also explore meditation more in Path 6.

Progressive muscle relaxation is also helpful. Starting with your feet, you contract and relax each part of the body as you progress up to the top of your head. Search Insighttimer.com for guided relaxation.

Cognitive behavioural therapy for insomnia

Cognitive behavioural therapy for insomnia (CBT-I) has been shown to improve sleep for many people. There are now versions available online and through apps (see resources). Some may be available free of charge, or they might be free with a referral from your GP. This is certainly something to investigate if sleep disturbance is persisting for a while. Or even just to gain new ideas for how to improve your sleep. Reputable versions are based on high quality research from leading sleep researchers, so this is definitely something to pursue to help you get a good night's sleep.

Shorten the night with sleep restriction therapy

If you have very poor-quality sleep, then contrary to what I said at the beginning of this milestone about giving yourself an 8-hour sleep opportunity, actually shortening your time in bed has also been shown to help.[53] Forcing yourself to go to bed later or to get up earlier can improve the quality of sleep, with a gradual lengthening of the time in bed as sleep quality improves. It can cause daytime sleepiness, which can be dangerous, but this is one of the few techniques that has been proven to help with longer-term insomnia. Michael Mosley explains the process in his book *Fast Asleep*. Speak to your GP first if you are thinking about trying sleep restriction therapy.

Magnesium

You may have read that magnesium is an important mineral for good sleep, so it might be helpful to read a bit more about magnesium's role in sleep to see if it could help you. You will find some articles from reputable sources on the internet.[54] Foods such as dark leafy greens, seeds, nuts, legumes and dark chocolate are rich in magnesium. You can also have a bath with Epsom salts, which contains magnesium and is absorbed through the skin. There are also a variety of magnesium supplements (in tablet and spray form), so if you think you want to take one do read around the subject rather than picking a supplement at random at the health shop or pharmacy. There are pros and cons to taking any supplement,[55] especially if you are taking any other medications (either prescribed or over-the-counter) or have any health conditions, so do speak to your pharmacist before taking any supplements. **That is very important and I can't emphasise it enough**. I hope the bold writing helps! Nothing is without some risk so it is important that you weigh it up for yourself.

Medications

Some medications can affect sleep, so do speak to your pharmacist if you suspect that something you are taking might be impacting on your sleep. Sleeping pills might be something you have considered taking if your sleep problems are persisting. Chronic insomnia is often described as a sleep problem that has lasted for more than three months,[56] but many people will have shorter-term sleep problems too. Whilst pills might be an obvious solution, they can often cause longer-term difficulties.[57] A number of attendees at my workshops on sleep have had long-term sleeping difficulties which they attribute to sleeping pills. There may well be times when sleeping pills are a helpful short-term support, but I would suggest you have a detailed discussion with your GP before taking them and read around the subject too. Try all of the other tips first and only use them as a last resort.

Napping

What about naps? Many societies embrace naps or afternoon siestas. If they work for you, great – go for it and enjoy them. Every now and again if I have had a very busy time and am feeling tired in the afternoon, I find a short nap very refreshing. Much of the advice around napping suggests not leaving it later than 3pm, and limiting it to 30 minutes maximum, but again find out what works for you. If napping doesn't disrupt your night-time sleep, then enjoy them, but I know that if I have a doze late in the evening, usually while watching the TV on the sofa (you can picture it I am sure), then it disrupts my sleep at about 4am. So I try really hard not to doze in the evening. If you are in danger of dozing in the few hours before bed, try doing something that engages your brain for a while like a crossword or number puzzle, or go out for a walk or do some yoga – anything that stops you nodding off before bedtime. I find that on the whole, if I am well rested and in good health, I don't feel tired until just before bedtime. If you find you regularly need naps, try to work out why, and make some changes to your lifestyle if at all possible. And get checked for any underlying health issues such as sleep apnoea, which is so dangerous if you are a driver and also has a longer-term impact on your health.

So hopefully by following some of this advice you will go off to sleep easily and sleep well all night. But what if you do tend to wake up in the middle of the night and can't go back to sleep? This is a very common problem, so don't think you are unusual if this happens to you. Different stages of life can impact on our ability to sleep and to stay asleep. Maybe you have a busy, stressful job, or young children or other caring duties. Maybe you have a health condition that is affecting you, or you are going through the menopause. A noisy neighbourhood may be keeping you awake at night, or you might have got into some unhealthy habits such as drinking alcohol every evening. Whatever your situation, maintaining your sleep throughout the night can be challenging at times.

I am sure you will have heard that there are different stages of sleep. Each night is made up of a number of sleep cycles, each of which lasts on average 90–120 minutes. Each cycle involves different phases: REM (rapid eye movement) and non-REM (NREM). As we fall asleep we go into the first stage of NREM, during which time we are easily awakened. Then we enter stage 2, which we can think of as light sleep. Next is stage 3, which is deep sleep. During this stage we are much harder to waken and our heart rate slows and our body temperature drops. It is in this stage of sleep that the body repairs and builds the immune system. Then we enter the REM phase, where we dream. We have longer deep sleep in the earlier part of the night and longer REM sleep in the later part of the night. At the end of each cycle we briefly wake up, but often that is not remembered in the morning. If you are someone who is conscious of waking in the night, then it is probably at this natural end to one of your sleep cycles. So waking in the night is a natural and normal thing to do, but it can be annoying if it means not being able to get back to sleep easily. So what can you try if you have woken up but can't get back to sleep?

Distract your busy mind

Often when we wake in the night our mind shifts into overdrive and we start to think worrying thoughts. They usually feel far more serious during the night than in the day for some reason! I think it is because during the day there might be actions you can take to solve them, or you have other things to do that distract you. If this sounds like you, try writing down what is on your mind and see if that helps. You can keep a notebook next to the bed. Listening to spoken radio or a podcast can act as a distraction, take your mind off your worries and help you get back to sleep.

Breathing techniques

Different types of breathing patterns can help you get back to sleep. Slow breathing engages the vagus nerve, part of the para-sympathetic nervous system, which acts to calm you. It is part of what is known as the 'rest and digest' system, which helps us to relax. In contrast, the sympathetic nervous system acts to alert us and get us ready for action and is also known as the 'flight, fight or freeze' response. Somehow the use of the term 'sympathetic' for the system that makes us likely to fight seems wrong. No wonder I was always confused by that during my biology lessons, including when I taught it. Apologies here to my former pupils!

A popular breathing practice is the 4-7-8 technique: breathe in for a count of 4, hold for 7, breathe out for 8 and repeat. Or 4-6: breathe in for 4, out for 6 and repeat. You will notice that they both have a longer exhale than inhale, which is calming.

Recently some research showed that 'cyclic sighing' (also called the 'physiological sigh') was one of the most effective breathing techniques for relaxation.[58] Dr Andrew Huberman is one of the neuroscientists who conducted this research, and you can find him demonstrating how to breathe in this way on the internet.[59] How it works is that you do a double inhale. You breathe in deeply through your nose, and when you think your lungs are fairly full you take an extra inhale, (Huberman describes it as sneaking a little extra air in) and then you breathe out slowly and repeat this for a few minutes. I use this if I am awake during the night, and I must say that for me it works really well – not all the time of course, as none of these strategies do, but it definitely helps to relax me to the right level to nod off again.

There have been a few books about breathing published in recent times and they detail some very interesting research about the importance of how we breathe. One aspect that interests me the most is the importance of breathing through the nose rather than through the mouth. James Nestor, in his book *Breath*, details the harmful effects of mouth breathing. He advocates putting a little strip of medical tape on the mouth to keep the lips together at night, to encourage nasal breathing. I have used this technique occasionally and find it very helpful to remind me to breathe through my nose. Just a small piece of micropore tape, about 5cm x 1cm, applied to the face just above and below the lips to gently keep them together works well, without feeling too restrictive or unpleasant. Nestor says the nose is for breathing and the mouth is for eating, so don't breathe through the mouth! I now try to breathe through my nose when running, whereas before reading his book I breathed through my mouth. Not always easy, but I am working on it. The benefits he describes from nasal breathing include better sleep, lower blood pressure, reduced anxiety, reduced allergies and much more.

Trying to stay awake

Strangely, it has been shown that trying to stay awake can help you go back to sleep.[60] This is another method that I have used, and it does often work. I know that it has worked for lots of my clients too. I keep my eyes open as I breathe in for 4, close my eyes as I breathe out for 6 and repeat. Eventually my eyelids feel heavy and I drop off to sleep.

Relax

Often it is our minds that don't feel relaxed, but what if it is your body that feels tense? You can try the progressive body relaxation exercise mentioned earlier. Or spend 10 minutes listening to a guided meditation, which can help you to relax.

Get up

Getting out of bed and doing something non-stimulating in a low light room, such as reading a book or magazine, can be helpful. You should then return to bed only when you feel really tired. This has been proven to work well and is recommended by many sleep researchers. Part of the theory behind this is that you don't want to associate your bed with lying awake tossing and turning, so if you have been awake for about 20 minutes without getting back to sleep, then leaving your bed to go elsewhere is advisable.

Impala time

I must admit that once I am in bed, I am not getting up until morning, whatever happens! I do love my bed. Instead, if I have been awake for a while, I adopt a technique a friend explained to me. As a child, if she was awake during the night, her mother (who was obviously very wise) would say to her, 'Don't worry; you are just having impala time.' This was on the basis that impalas are a type of antelope that rarely sleep. So now if I am awake for a while, I snuggle down in my cosy bed and try to turn my thoughts to gratitude for all I have –and I enjoy my 'impala time'.

Bathroom visits

At my sleep workshops, one of the most complained about problems with sleep is the need to visit the bathroom during the night. The name for night-time peeing is nocturia. It becomes more common as we age and there can be some underlying health reasons for it. Unfortunately, menopause in women[61] and enlarged prostate[62] in men are two common reasons for this happening as we age, but do check with your doctor if you notice a change in your ability to sleep through the night because you wake up to use the bathroom, just in case there is some other cause. Not drinking too much close to bedtime can help, as can avoiding caffeine and alcohol.

I hope some of these tips will work for you if your sleep needs improving, but of course nothing works for everyone, so you do need to personalise the advice. And don't worry if you don't bounce out of bed first thing in the morning as it is normal to have up to half an hour of 'sleep inertia'. This is the groggy feeling you may get on waking. The important thing to consider is how your energy levels are during the day. If you are having trouble with sleeping on a regular basis, do speak to your doctor to rule out any underlying causes such as an illness or sleep apnoea. Plus, there are so many other conditions that affect sleep which are not covered in this book, such as jet lag, night-shift working, nightmares and sleep walking. There is help out there, so do seek help if there is something else bothering you that affects your sleep – don't suffer in silence.

And remember, sleep benefits all our biological functions and resets our brains and bodies overnight, so give it the priority it deserves. Sweet dreams!

Sandra's story

Path 5 of the *Positive Paths to Wellbeing* course really resonated with me, especially the section on staying active. It emphasised the need to look after four elements of my physical health: flexibility, aerobic fitness, balance and strength. I had recently had a bit of a scare when I tried to get myself out of the sea when on holiday in Majorca. There was a ladder to help me out but I really struggled to pull myself up onto it, and I realised that the strength in my arms had got rather weak as I had got older. It was quite a shock. It made me realise I wanted and needed to keep healthy into old age. Marie saying she wanted to be able to lift her own suitcase into the overhead locker in the plane really resonated with me. So, spurred on by this, I have added in a variety of different activities to help build back my strength. I bought some dumbbells and started to lift those. I joined a step class, and another gym class for balance and strength and now go to these on a regular basis. I think I took my strength and fitness for granted when I was younger but that wake-up call in the sea in Majorca has really changed how I approach my physical health. I find that there is also a mental challenge in my step class when I have to coordinate all the different routines – definitely a workout for the mind too. A win-win! *Path 5 – Look after my body* is now a key focus of my life.

Path 6
Look after my mind

'You can't stop the waves but you can learn to surf.'
Jon Kabat-Zinn

6:A – Be kind to myself

Most of the subjects we have covered in the previous five paths will have an impact on your mental health, from your relationships with others, to how good your diet is, to how well you sleep. But in this path, we are going to look in a bit more detail at what we can do to help our minds or our mental wellbeing. We started to think about our mental wellbeing in *Nurture my relationship with myself* in Path 3, so do go back and revisit that path if you have forgotten the content and your answers to the questions.

I often think about how I feel in terms of a Scale of Wellbeing, which you can see on page 151. I think of the neutral position as feeling fine or ok, neither happy nor miserable. And this might be how you feel much of the time – just fine. But hopefully there are times when you feel up in the positive zone. And this can change on an hourly or daily basis. If you are anything like me, then life is full of ups and downs and we simply couldn't live our lives, or even want to live our lives, at +10 all of the time.

Scale of Wellbeing

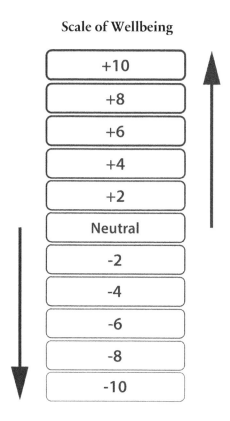

If we have the normal human responses to the events that happen to us, then we will experience joy, sadness, grief, guilt, anger, excitement, embarrassment, love and the full range of human emotions. We might be happily in the positive zone when we hear of a very sad situation like the death of a loved one and we are immediately plunged down into the negative zone. Or we might be feeling negative because we have been made redundant and then we find out we have landed a great new job and we are feeling positive again. These are major life events, but small events can also change our mood instantly, such as a sharp word from a loved one or colleague, or discovering a flat tyre as you jump in the car to head to the airport for your holiday. As I said, life is full of ups and downs, so have a think about where you are on the scale the majority of the time. If you are not happy with your answer, then the guidance in this book should help you to make changes that will move you up the scale.

If you feel that you are living in the negative zone most of the time, it is really important to get help. Remember that you are not alone; it's likely other people have suffered similar experiences to you and described their journey in books, podcasts, websites or through charities – and you may find these things resonate with you, helping you move towards the positive zone on the scale. Most importantly, if your mental health feels really negative, please do seek help. There is help available. You might start by going to your GP, but also seek out those resources where you can learn from others in a similar situation. Just choose carefully and make sure they are from reputable sources. You know what the internet is like! People do recover from periods of low mental health and there are techniques and therapies that do help, so never suffer in silence – seek help immediately from a trusted source. It might be a family member or friend, or a professional such as your GP, or a charity such as The Samaritans. It breaks my heart to hear of someone who died by suicide when I know that it might have been possible for them to get help that would have improved their mental wellbeing. Do have a look at the list of resources at the back of the book for other organisations that can help and take that first step and contact them.

It is also important to recognise that we all have mental health all of the time; it is the level, positive or negative, that is important. I sometimes hear of someone being described as 'they have mental health' when what is meant is that they are struggling with their mental health at the present time. As I said we all have mental health all of the time in the same way as we all have physical health all of the time. Sometimes good, sometimes not so good. Some people have negative levels for significant periods of time and need specialist help, but we can all use some help in managing the times when we are lower down the scale. This path is going to discuss techniques that have been shown to help improve mental wellbeing and move you up the scale, so do see if some of them appeal to you and perhaps give them a try.

Modern life can sometimes seem like a conveyor belt of tasks that never end. There are so many opportunities available to us that we simply can't do everything. Do you remember reading that in *Manage my time* in Path 2? Through social media we are bombarded with endless information about what others are doing, which can make us feel inadequate. Maybe during the time of the pandemic you managed to slow down a bit, but even then you might still have felt under pressure to do more with your downtime, such as become a brilliant baker! I seem to remember lots of recipes for banana bread being shared around. This path is going to look at some techniques that might slow down the conveyor belt and move you up the Scale of Wellbeing.

Comparison

In Path 3 I mentioned becoming your own best friend. Have you managed to do that? Have you tried to be a supportive friend to yourself, one who helps you learn from life and from your mistakes rather than one who is hard on you? One of the reasons we are often so hard on ourselves is because we compare ourselves to others. And this can bring a feeling of inferiority or indeed sometimes superiority, neither of which is going to lead to a happy, calm attitude to life. Before we go any further have a go at answering the questions below.

1. How have you implemented the concept of being your own best friend from Path 3?
2. Who do you compare yourself with on a regular basis? They could be people you know or people from the media. Include people who you compare yourself with favourably and unfavourably.

Comparing ourselves to others can lead to negative feelings, but remember that we are often only seeing one aspect of someone else's life. Ask yourself what benefit you are getting out of this comparison. Is it moving you towards the life you truly want? Sometimes the answer will be yes – after all we learn a lot from other people, and analysing some aspect of another person's success or accomplishments can spur us on to learn new skills and try new challenges. Other times we know that comparing ourselves to others is not helping us. If it is demotivating, or negatively impacts how you feel, then try to be more aware of when you are doing it. Comparison is a natural part of human behaviour.[1] But do try to question the impact it has on you, and if it has a negative impact, work out how you can change that. Maybe you might use social media less, or you might find writing about it in a journal can help you gain perspective. Talking to friends might help with getting a new perspective too. So again, be your own best friend, be self-aware and use comparison wisely. After all, you are a totally unique individual, so why would you expect to be the same as someone else? Let's all celebrate being different.

Reframing

Another way to be kind to yourself is to see things from different perspectives. A shorthand for this is to 'reframe'. Let me give you an example. I was coaching someone who was going for an interview, and they got through to the second stage, but they didn't get the job. Understandably they were disappointed as it was something they had set their heart on. We talked about the experience of the process and looked at the learning that came from it. A number of learning points were clear once we had analysed the situation. They had revamped their CV, made a connection with the new company, got interview experience and demonstrated their ambition to their current workplace. There were clear benefits from the process, even if they had not achieved their ultimate goal. They also received some feedback and found out they had come a close second and that the company had been very impressed with them. When things don't work out exactly as you want, can you look at the experience in a different way? Identify all of the goals you had and not just the main one, learn from the experience and judge it in a more rounded way – again, be kind to yourself. Is there a situation that you need to reframe so that you can learn and grow from it?

Self-compassion

Being kind to yourself is not about self-pity or self-indulgence. It is not a green light to give up and lie on the sofa, eating from a bucket of ice cream and watching rubbish on the TV. Instead, it is about acknowledging you are human, that life is not perfect and neither are you, and then deciding what you want to do that links you back to the important things in your life – right back to *Path 1 – Clarify what is important to me*. Research has shown that self-compassion is one of the best ways to develop resilience and coping strategies, and that it builds mental and physical health; it really does work. Take a look at the work of Dr Kirsten Neff,[2] a leading researcher on self-compassion, to find out more. So when you find that you are being hard on yourself, keep asking what your kindest friend would say, and then take that to heart. Life is tough enough without beating ourselves up over natural human behaviour.

6:B – Live in the moment

This section focuses on negative thoughts and emotions and explains some helpful techniques for dealing with them, but it does ask you to remember some negative thoughts in order to try out the techniques. Consider if this is something that is right for you at the moment, and if you feel that you are not in the right frame of mind just now, move on to *6:C Find time for yourself*.

I don't know about you, but my mind is always pulling me into the future or back into the past. Sometimes this is very deliberate and conscious on my part. I might be busy planning something to do with work, or a holiday, or maybe what to cook for dinner. And sometimes I love thinking about the past; lovely times I have had with family and friends or learning from something that I did recently. I might be thinking about a coaching client and reflecting on my session with them in order to help my understanding of what was helpful and not so helpful.

A lot of the time my mind goes to the future or the past but I don't seem to have consciously chosen the thoughts. Does this sound familiar to you? One clear example to me is if I wake in the night and struggle to go back to sleep because my mind is racing with thoughts – sometimes positive ones and sometimes worrying ones. If I had a switch, I would most certainly turn the thoughts off so I could go straight back to sleep.

Negative thoughts

If you find that your mind often has negative thoughts playing over and over, I'm afraid to inform you that this is completely normal. Humans survived and evolved as a species because they were great at watching out for danger – keeping an eye out for the sabre-toothed tiger lurking in the bushes! So whilst we don't have to watch out for tigers wanting to turn us into dinner, we are still on the lookout for anything that threatens us – and that can be something a loved one says to us, a post on social media or critical thoughts in which we compare ourselves to others. Do take a few minutes to think about how much time you spend in past and future thoughts.

You may be wondering if there is anything we can do to help with negative thoughts. I have studied Acceptance and Commitment Therapy (ACT), which I use in my coaching, and I am going to introduce you to some ACT techniques for dealing with difficult thoughts and feelings.

Observing thoughts

Can you think of a negative thought that pops into your mind unbidden on a regular basis? Maybe it is a worry about children, work, or the future, or a criticism of yourself. The next time that you find yourself thinking this particular thought, I want you to notice it. Let's say the thought is a worry about a public speaking engagement you have coming up. Your brain might be saying, 'I'm going to be so nervous and mess it up.'

Now picture two parts of your brain: the part that is doing the thinking, and another part of the brain that is able to notice that you are thinking that particular thought. This is known as metacognition. So you might be able to catch yourself at some point and say, 'Ah ha, I am having the thought that I'm going to mess up the presentation.' Now as soon as you catch yourself noticing that thought, you can name it ('Here is the messed-up-presentation thought again'), or label it as a story ('Here is the messed-up-presentation story') because that is what it is – a story. You have no idea whether or not it will happen. You might mess up the presentation, but you might do a great job; it depends on many factors, such as the amount of preparation and practice you put in and what happens on the day in the time leading up to the presentation. So, the next time you identify you are worrying about something, can you notice the worrying thoughts and then name them? Give your story a title. Accept that this is how our minds work and then focus on doing something that moves your life in the direction you want it to go – think all the way back to Path 1 when you clarified what was important to you. That might be going for a walk, reading a good book, having a chat with a loved one; it's anything that enriches your life. In the case of the messed-up-presentation story, the best thing might be to focus on practising your presentation and minimising the chances of it going wrong. *2:C Manage my time* can help you get organised so that you can achieve this goal.

Write it down

Another action you can take which has been shown to be effective for dealing with difficult thoughts is to write about them. Spend 15 minutes either writing by hand or typing on the computer. You can then choose to keep it or get rid of the writing. I use this technique for when I have been dwelling on something, and it really helps me. I sometimes have quite a rant! I type away without concerning myself with spelling or punctuation and then at the end I just delete it. We can't turn off our thoughts but we can recognise them for what they are – words or stories in our head.

But you might say, 'What if the thoughts are true'. In ACT, whether the thoughts are true or not isn't important. The crucial question to ask is whether this thought is helpful. Will it help you in the life you want to live? If it is helpful, then pay attention to it and learn from it, but if it isn't, then focus on something that will help you live the life you want.

There are lots of great techniques in ACT for dealing with difficult thoughts, so if this intrigues you, why not have a read of *The Happiness Trap* by Russ Harris. I use these techniques in my coaching and they are so powerful. It is something I think everyone should be taught from a young age.

Dealing with emotions

What if we are more troubled by our emotions, those powerful feelings that show up in our body? Here ACT can help too. As someone who studied and taught biology, although many years ago now, I am fascinated by how the body works and, in particular, how our mind impacts on our body and vice versa; you could argue they are one and the same thing. The brain is indeed part of the body! As a human being you will be more than familiar with the changing emotions that we can feel. As mentioned earlier, one minute you can be happy, then you hear some sad news, or even just conjure up a thought, and you can be moved into a completely different emotional state. Or you might be feeling a bit low, you hear some positive news and it lifts your mood instantly. We are generally not too keen on the more negative emotions and people often try different ways to get rid of them, such as comfort eating, alcohol or drugs, excess exercise or just trying to 'think positively'. Regardless of whether we like negative feelings or not, as human beings we will feel this range of emotions throughout our lives, so we need to learn how to cope with the more difficult emotions. Again, ACT can come to the rescue and help us to recognise what we are experiencing and how to make peace with our emotions.

Expansion

Now I want you to bring to mind a slightly uncomfortable emotion, nothing too heavy, but just something you are not too keen on – maybe some embarrassment at something you did in the past. And just sit with this emotion for a few seconds, then answer the following questions.

1. Where can you feel the emotion in your body?
2. What does it look like?
3. Can you imagine it as an object?
4. What shape is it?
5. What colour is it?
6. Is it heavy or light?
7. Is the surface shiny or dull?
8. Is the surface smooth or does it have a texture or bits protruding from it?
9. Is it moving or still?

I want you to breathe in slowly, and as you breathe out, I want you to picture your breath starting to surround the object. At first it's just a tiny bit of air, but with each exhale a bit more air starts to surround the object. As you continue to breathe, you can imagine the air around the object growing bigger and bigger. So just sit with this for as long as you like, allowing the air around the object to grow and grow.

How did you find that? Strange, I am sure. After all we don't normally picture our emotions as objects in our body. For me, embarrassment appears as a blue, fluffy cloud-like object just under my ribs on the right of my body. Anxiety is a heavy, smooth, silver dumbbell just over my heart. I had never tried to picture my emotions like this before learning about ACT, so don't be surprised if you find this difficult or impossible at the moment. But do try again the next time you feel a genuine emotion rather than the more artificial experience of reading this book and trying to conjure one up from the past.

The aim of this visualisation is not to get rid of the emotion or the object, but just to sit with it, in a way that is slightly different from normal. It is most important not to try to get rid of it, as acceptance of our emotions is very important in managing them – hence the acceptance part of 'Acceptance and Commitment Therapy'. The emotion and object might change as you focus your breath in this way, but getting rid of them is not the purpose. You are learning to sit with your emotions. I, perhaps rather simplistically, think of emotions as being caused by messages that pass along my nerves, making my body produce hormones, and that there is nothing permanent about them – they come and they go. It is not like losing a limb, which is permanent; emotions are transient. If you think about all of the different emotions you will have experienced over the last few days, I hope that the transience of emotions is something that rings true for you. This technique is known as 'expansion' in ACT and can be very helpful when you experience emotions that you find hard to manage. With practice you can learn to picture them, to breathe around them and to allow them to be. Know that they are a part of being a human being and that they come and go – not always as quickly as we might like, but they can be bearable, even interesting, when we learn to accept them. I so wish I had known about these techniques when I was struggling with post-natal depression. Fortunately I did know about them when I experienced anxiety as part of the perimenopause and used these techniques frequently. I would also say to myself 'It is just your nerves and hormones trying to stay young!'

Being mindful

ACT is an example of a mindfulness-based therapy. You have almost certainly heard of mindfulness. It has become more popular recently as it has been shown to improve wellbeing.[3] I have first-hand experience of this as I was involved with a mindfulness-based stress reduction programme in the NHS[4] that had some really profound benefits for the participants. When people talk about mindfulness, they are usually talking about mindfulness meditation. There is an eight-week programme of mindfulness meditation that has been shown to help with depression. It is now recommended by the National Institute for Health and Care Excellence (NICE)[5] in the UK. I have given the details of a mindfulness book that covers this programme in the resources at the end of the book as well as details of an online version of the course.[6] Many people start their own programme of mindfulness meditation using apps such as Headspace or Calm. It is definitely worth investigating these apps to see if they could be helpful for you.

But mindfulness is not just about meditation; mindfulness is also about being more in the present moment, being aware of what you are doing right now and not thinking or dwelling on the past or worrying about the future. So even if you aren't interested in trying out mindfulness meditation, you can practise placing your attention on the present moment, getting totally absorbed in what you are doing. That might be eating slowly and thoughtfully, really noticing the taste of your food rather than mindlessly wolfing down a whole packet of crisps without savouring each bite. Or it might be noticing the flowers, buds and leaves on the plants when you are out walking. Or maybe it's noticing the view when you are driving, rather than having your mind elsewhere and thinking about the past or the future. A shower in the morning is a great way to start the day mindfully. Rather than thinking about what you need to do that day, slow down, wash yourself with care and notice the feel of water on your skin.

Why not take a few moments now to think about when you are most mindful? What activities do you do that hold you firmly in the present moment and stop you thinking about the past or the future, or stop you criticising yourself or worrying? I know for me getting engrossed in a really good book grips me and stops me thinking about anything else. I am partial to a number puzzle too. Maybe you have a hobby that does that. Or maybe there are certain people who you love to be with, and you give them all your attention when you are with them. Maybe some form of exercise is mindful for you. So why not write these down and plan to ensure they are regular features in your life?

Focused breathing

I mentioned cyclic sighing (or physiological sigh) in *5:C Sleep well*, and this is good for bringing you back to the present moment. It can also help during the day if you are feeling a bit stressed. Spend a few minutes doing a few rounds of cyclic sighing. I like to do it and smile at the same time which, for me, boosts the effectiveness. Breathe in deeply through your nose, and when you think your lungs are fairly full take an extra inhale, then breathe out slowly and repeat this for a few minutes. You can use this any time you feel a bit tense, stressed or anxious. You may also find some other types of focused breathing help you. Maybe breathing in for a count of 4 and out for 6 slowly. Or breathing in for 4 and then slowly breathe out as if you are blowing through a straw, making your exhale really slow and long.

Meditation

As we finish the *Live in the moment* milestone of Path 6, let's take a few minutes to do a guided meditation. If you already have an app, select your favourite meditation. If you have never tried guided meditation before, have a look on the internet for one that appeals to you. Insighttimer.com has an extensive range. Alternatively, you can sit still with your eyes closed for a few minutes and just focus on your breath, as detailed in the next paragraph. One of the reasons that many meditations focus on the breath is that it is very handy as we always have it with us. Slowing the breath also calms us down by engaging the para-sympathetic nervous system (as mentioned before in *5:C Sleep well*). If you don't want to focus on the breath, as not everyone likes that, then just tap gently on your leg or hand instead and focus on that. You only need to start off with a few minutes, but it will give you an idea of what it is like. You do need to practise regularly, as with any skill. If you start with a few minutes a couple of times a day, you should find that it becomes much easier and that you can use it when you are feeling a bit stressed. It brings a bit of peace into your daily life. So have a read of the next paragraph and then put the book down and spend a few minutes being mindful.

Guided meditation instructions

Sit comfortably, feet flat on the floor, back supported but relaxed, hands in your lap. Gently relax your eyes, or close them if you prefer, and take a slow breath in and out. Don't try to change your breath in any way, just bring your attention to your breath. Picture it going in and out as your chest rises and falls. Notice where your attention is. Is it on your breath or some thought that has carried you away from your breath? Getting carried away by a thought is completely natural, so when you notice that your mind has wandered, just return your attention to your breath; each time your mind wanders, very gently bring it back. It is perfectly normal for your mind to wander off a hundred times, so don't be annoyed with yourself; just silently say, 'Thank you, mind,' and gently return to the in-and-out flow of breath. After focusing on your breath for a short while, move your attention to the sounds around you, then gently bring your attention back to your breath. After a few breaths, turn your attention to your body on the chair, then to your feet on the ground, then to your hands in your lap. Scan your body, starting with the top of your head and gradually working down to the soles of your feet. Note any areas of tension or discomfort or calm. Again, after a short while, bring your attention back to your breath once more. Relax your shoulders, slow your breathing and then gradually come back to the awareness of your room and open your eyes. Read the instructions once more, then put down the book and give it a go.

How did you find that? If it is your first time, you will probably have found it quite strange, but research has shown that regularly practising mindful meditation can bring benefits to your mental wellbeing.[7] How could you incorporate a regular mindfulness meditation practice into your life? I must admit that it is something I find difficult to do, despite my best intentions, but I do know that when I can make time for it regularly I am more easily able to relax, so it is definitely something I am working on. I have bought a lovely beanbag for meditation (very retro), and I am now finding that I do meditate more as a result.

So that brings us to the end of this milestone. I hope that some of these techniques will be useful for you as you navigate the emotional journey that is every human's life.

Learning how to live more in the moment and not in the past or the future can have real, tangible benefits for your mental wellbeing.

6:C – Find time for myself

The third milestone of Path 6 is all about finding time for yourself. Let's revisit the Scale of Wellbeing from milestone 6:A and examine in more detail what lifts us up and what moves us down. Have a look at the scale and think how you have generally been feeling over the last few months. What would be your most common score? I know this is not very scientific, but I find it can be helpful to recognise if you have been generally in the positive zone, or fairly neutral (where life is fine or ok), or generally in the negative zone (where life is not great and needs to change). Can you pinpoint what is causing you to feel that way? Take a moment to have a think about what has been happening for you recently.

Did you find it easy or difficult to pinpoint the cause of how you have been feeling? Maybe work is going really well, or you have been doing plenty of exercise and this is having a positive impact. Or maybe there is some sadness in your life, or some dissatisfaction. Maybe this is how you almost always feel because you do not vary very much. Or maybe you have no idea why you feel the way you do, and that is also fine.

Now I would like to go back to the Wheel of Wellbeing that you focused on in Path 1. Work around the Wheel and identify things in each area that lift you up, moving you into the positive zone, or take you down into the negative zone. For example in the fitness segment, getting out for a walk might be uplifting, while being hunched over a computer all day with few breaks and no exercise might bring you down. Think about each area and also be conscious of whether there are any activities that lift you up in the short term, only to take you down in the long term. Alcohol might be an example here: a glass of wine might relax you and help you to unwind; a bottle on the other hand will probably lead to a bad night's sleep, a hangover and a wasted day. So make sure you put some detail into your list.

I am sure you will have lots of ideas about what lifts you up. I am going to mention a few here, and you will find a longer list at the end of this milestone.

Wellbeing activities
Obviously exercise, eating well and sleeping well will help to improve how you feel. Not drinking too much alcohol and staying hydrated will be top of your mind now you have just completed Path 5.

Spending time with good friends and having a laugh are great for your wellbeing. Even just smiling has been shown to increase mood by tricking your brain. It might seem that you only smile when you are happy, but you can smile first and this makes you feel happier. Seems strange but it does work. Why not give it a try it now? Just curl up the corners of your mouth! ☺

Being outside in nature has been shown to have a positive effect on mood, so try to build some time in nature into your everyday life, even just a short walk can help. Getting a short walk first thing in the morning is a great habit to get into. I mentioned it in *5:C Sleep well* too, as it sets your body clock and makes it easier to sleep at night – a double win.

What about hobbies? Getting really absorbed in something interesting has also been shown to boost wellbeing. When something really absorbs us, we get into so-called 'flow' or 'being in the zone'. (I will cover this again in Path 8.) I know for me if I don't get the chance to do something creative every now and again, I really notice that it brings me down the Scale of Wellbeing. Maybe art or music or reading lifts you up, or maybe puzzles like crosswords or Sudoku.

Helping others has also been shown to increase wellbeing, whether that is something informal like popping in to check on your elderly neighbour, or something more organised like volunteering in the local charity shop. So have a think about what you can do to help others.

Establishing a daily gratitude practice can be another way to improve your wellbeing. Research has shown that being grateful is a proven way to feel better.[8] Writing a list of things you are grateful for at the end of each day can be a really positive daily practice. I start each work day writing three things I am grateful for in my daily planner. It is a lovely, positive way to start my day. Many people think of a few things they are grateful for last thing at night as they are going off to sleep. In a world where bad news on the TV might be one of the last things we see before going to bed (why do they have the news at 10pm?), a few moments to appreciate the good things in our lives can be a gentle way to wind down.

Something that might surprise you that has been proven to help improve mood: a hot bath. It is thought that it helps reset circadian rhythms, so a bath is maybe something else worth considering. In a piece of research, two hot baths a week were effective in improving mood in patients with depression.[9] Maybe one of the reasons hot tubs are rather popular, they lift you up the Scale of Wellbeing.

Having a hug is a well-known stress reducer.[10] The hormone oxytocin is released during a cuddle and can be very calming, depending on who is hugging you! You can also try hugging yourself and it might even help with sending you off to sleep. Why not try hugging yourself right now. Go on, have a big squeeze and slow down your breath. See how much calmer you feel.

There is a list at the end of this milestone of more ideas for activities that can lift you up the Scale of Wellbeing, but remember that it is important to work out what is right for you. We are all different, so the activities that lift us up will vary. You may have a friend who loves wild camping, which is your idea of hell, and you might love a luxurious spa, which your friend hates. Watching a murder mystery on TV might be just the thing to relax you and to help you to be mindful, but for someone else that might cause them stress. It is important to be curious about what works for you and know yourself.

Saying no

My final thought before we leave this path is that sometimes in order to find time for ourselves, we need to say no. No to things that we recognise are not good for us, or to things that we don't have time for, and that are not high on our list of priorities. Remember back in Path 2 the simple scale of 'important' and 'not important'? In order to find time for ourselves we have to be clear about what is important to us, and good mental wellbeing should be high up that scale. So you may need to gently say no to some things. Maybe postpone them to another time or suggest someone else does them. Or maybe it is not about saying no to someone else, but to ourselves. Saying no to spending too much time on social media, or to another glass of wine or packet of crisps, or no to tidying up after children who can do their own tidying. Not so sure I really cracked that one! Have a think about the following questions.

1. What do you say yes to when you would prefer to say no? Think about saying yes/no to others and think about saying yes/no to yourself.
2. Why do you think you say yes?
3. If appropriate, how could you (gently) say no the next time? You may want to revisit the list of ways to say no at the end of *2:C Manage my time*.
4. How could you find more time for the activities that lift you up the Scale of Wellbeing?

It isn't selfish to prioritise time for yourself. Without looking after yourself, you can't look after others. Or you might be able to for a while, but eventually you may find everything becomes a bit overwhelming. Have you heard the expression 'you can't pour from an empty cup'? Work out what fills your cup and make time in your diary for those activities.

Getting help

There are so many different challenges that people face with their mental health that this path only touches on a few ideas for supporting good mental health. If you feel that your mental health could be better or you have a diagnosed condition, I hope that you are able to seek out the help that is available from the NHS or other organisations. Charities like Mind are great starting points for getting support, and there are also many books written about different mental health conditions including advice on how to move up the Scale of Wellbeing. A good book to start with is *Why Has Nobody Told Me This Before?* by Dr Julie Smith. She also shares short videos on her social media channels. I love her straightforward approach and thoroughly recommend her work to you.

As we end Path 6, I hope that you have been inspired by the idea of being kind to yourself and being more mindful, that you will take some precious time for yourself and, most importantly, that if you do need support to improve your mental health, you seek it out. There are people waiting to help who understand what you are going through.

Wellbeing activities

- Hobbies
- Crafting
- Reading
- Puzzles
- Drawing/art
- Music/singing
- Exercise
- Sports
- Being out in nature
- Gardening
- Having a laugh
- Helping others
- Dancing
- Writing in a journal
- Digital down time
- Comedy
- Hot baths
- Yoga
- Cuddles
- Intimacy
- Meditating
- Stroking a pet
- Praying
- Self-compassion
- Mindfulness
- Learning

Anything else that lifts you up and is good for both your short-term and long-term wellbeing.

Anne's story

I took the *Positive Paths to Wellbeing* course at a stressful time in my life. I had recently had some family bereavements and also some problems with my health. I found *Path 6 – Look after my mind* particularly helpful. I had not come across Acceptance and Commitment Therapy before, but I found that when I could catch myself having repeated negative thoughts, I started to be able to label them as a 'story'. A story that I could not change and that was not helpful. I then found that the circles of control from *Path 2 – Take personal responsibility* helped me to focus on what I could control. When I caught myself in one of these negative stories, I started to say to myself, 'Ah, here is the stress story,' and then make myself focus on what I could do that would lift me up the Scale of Wellbeing. For me, that was painting or gardening. Art painting, not the decorating kind! I still have times when I get lost in the stress story but I am so much better at catching myself and turning my focus to something I can control. Getting outside to garden or painting a picture always lifts me up.

Path 7
Develop positive habits

'We first make our habits, then our habits make us.'
John Dryden

7:A – Make small changes

The paths that we have travelled so far have focused on some of the key areas of life. In this next path we consider how we can get into good habits, so that we can take action in each of these key areas. Much of what we have been covering so far has been about making small changes, but it can be very hard for even small changes to stick, so this path looks at how to embed those changes into your everyday life.

A number of years ago I read a book called *The Slight Edge* by Jeff Olson and it had a really profound impact on me. Jeff emphasised that it was all the little things that you do every day that add up, and often we don't notice those little things until much further down the line, maybe months or even years later. Often the difference between good health and poor health is the result of small changes, such as eating a few more vegetables at dinner or short bursts of activity each day. And often we don't notice these things when we are young, but as we get older we start to see and appreciate how our daily habits add up, for better or worse. Below is a visual representation of that idea.

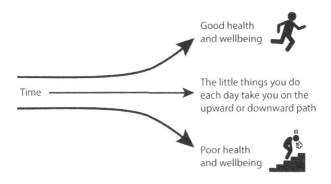

Imagine eating a doughnut every day. It's probably not going to have a big impact on you in a week, or maybe even in a month, but eating food that is high in sugar and fat and low in nutrients and fibre, over a long period of time, can increase the risk of being overweight which can eventually lead to metabolic syndrome,[1] Type 2 diabetes[2] and heart disease,[3] and then it's hard to undo the damage. Imagine you are starting a new exercise regime. If you are anything like me you will hope to wake up the next day with strong muscles, a six pack and full of energy, but instead you've probably got some aching muscles and are wondering if you're going to be able to keep going with your new regime. But if you stick with it over time, you will find that your muscles don't hurt any more, you are getting stronger, you have more energy, your clothes fit better, and all the activities of daily life are so much easier. But I know how easy it is to give up when you don't see results quickly, which is probably why Jeff Olsen's message had such a profound effect on me and really helped me to stick to my daily exercise regime and other daily habits. So the first milestone of Path 7 focuses on making small changes and finding ways to make new habits stick.

One of the important things to note about habits is that they occur subconsciously. It has been estimated that almost half[4] of the things we do each day are in fact habits. We don't need to use any higher thinking; we just get on and do them. Getting up, showering, eating, snacking, checking our phones, even driving – these things are often done on automatic pilot. They are part of our everyday routines. Fortunately, we do have the ability to look at our habits and to make changes if we realise they are not helping us live the life we want to lead. However, it is not easy, as you will surely know if you have ever tried to start a new good habit or break an old bad one. Before we go any further, I want you to think about your current good habits. Make a list and then consider what helps you to stick to them. I am sure you will have lots of good habits!

A few years ago I started to hear more about the health benefits of a dip in cold water.[5] Whilst there may be some debate about whether cold water is good for you, one of the theories is that the cold water is stressful to the body, and regular exposure to this stress makes us more able to cope with other stresses. In our modern society we might go from a warm home into a warm car into a warm workplace, and we no longer experience the variations our ancestors experienced. Although you may not have to think back far to remember it yourself. Growing up we didn't have central heating in our draughty old house and I clearly remember the ice on the inside of my bedroom window in the winter. Now my remotely controlled thermostat means I never have to experience a cold house, and believe you me I am very grateful, as I realise that for many people the cost of heating means they regularly have a cold house in the winter.

So back to my cold-water exposure. The easiest way to get this on a regular basis is to turn the water to cold at the end of a warm shower. The first time I tried this I was pleasantly surprised about how it felt. Admittedly I turned the temperature down gradually and did not stay in for long, but I certainly felt more energised afterwards. I was sold on this as a new habit right from this first experience. But as always with new habits, it can be hard to make them stick. I soon forgot about it despite finding it a pleasant (or should that be 'interesting') experience. But I read a lot of wellbeing research, and cold-water exposure appeared again with lots of claims about health benefits, so I restarted my habit. I was determined to stick with it this time, and so far, so good – it seems to have become a set part of my day. I must admit that I sometimes go for cool rather than cold, and some days I stay under longer than others.

Do be careful if you are planning to start cold-water exposure and check with your doctor first if you have any health conditions or take any medication.

Minimum viable habit

Having some flexibility but setting a minimum expectation works for me. I think of this as my 'minimum viable habit' (MVH). You may have heard of 'minimum viable product', when new products are being developed, and I apply that to my healthy habits. What is the minimum I can do to make it worthwhile, so that even on the days when I don't feel in the mood I know I can do this minimum amount? With my morning exercise habit that I mentioned earlier, my MVH is a set of arm exercises and a set of leg exercises (such as a few push-ups and squats). I can nearly always find the time or the enthusiasm for that small amount, even on very busy days. Note I did say 'nearly'!

Now I know I have mentioned this many times throughout the book already, but I really want to emphasise how important it is to recognise that the small things can and do make a difference. Even this MVH makes a difference. In Dr Chatterjee's book *Feel Better in 5*, he focuses on three five-minute activities per day – yes, just 15 minutes in total – which can have a profound impact on your life.

Establishing habits

Maybe you have read that a new habit takes 21 days to form, or maybe you have heard three months or some other timescale, but personally I don't believe any of them as I know for me the timescale very much depends on what I am trying to start. Some habits have quickly become a new part of my life and others have taken a lot longer to embed. There are also habits I have had for years that I then stop, so be curious about how starting a new habit works for you.

My morning exercise routine took many months to become something I did at least four or five days a week, and it didn't seem to make a big difference to my fitness at first, but who knows how my physical health would be now if I hadn't started it. Maybe I would be suffering with a sore back, maybe I would struggle to carry heavy shopping, maybe I would be heavier and less fit and then less able to go for a walk in the hills or do a long-distance walk. Since embedding a new habit is not going to be easy, you want to make sure you put your energy and focus into what is really important to you. So I would like you to have a think about what ideas you have had for change as you have read through the book, and see if you can identify just one or two new habits that, if you managed to make them a part of your daily life, would make the biggest difference and would be worth the effort.

The Habit Cycle

How do you go about introducing a new habit? If you look into the studies of habits, you will probably find a version of the habit cycle.[6] The cycle starts with some type of reminder – you might think of this as a cue or trigger – which prompts the response that leads to the reward. Let me use brushing your teeth as an example, as you will see in the diagram on page 182. The reminder, or cue, to brush your teeth might be finishing your shower, so you do it every day at the same time. The response is the action of brushing your teeth and the reward is that you have a clean, minty-fresh mouth. You don't even have to think about it, as it is just part of your regular routine.

The Habit Cycle

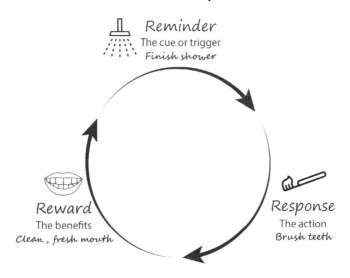

Reminder
The cue or trigger
Finish shower

Response
The action
Brush teeth

Reward
The benefits
Clean , fresh mouth

We can use this reminder-response-reward cycle to set up a new habit. One of the first things to consider is how you will get the necessary reminder. So often the reason that I have not done something I had planned to do was that 'I simply forgot!' Nothing reminded me to do it. Therefore linking a new habit to an old habit is one of the easiest ways to trigger the reminder. If, for example, you wanted to start flossing your teeth on a daily basis, the reminder would be brushing your teeth. The response would be carrying out the flossing and the reward would be a cleaner mouth. The behaviour scientist and author of *Tiny Habits*, B J Fogg, suggests making the new habit as tiny as possible to get you started, so in this case he would suggest just flossing one tooth. It seems a little crazy to think about flossing just one tooth, but if you can break down more overwhelming habits into tiny ones, you're much more likely to get started. Then once you've started, you'll probably do more – you'll probably do two teeth or maybe even go wild and do your whole mouth! This is similar to my minimum viable habit that I mentioned earlier. Dental health is often an overlooked area of our health. It is not just to make sure we keep all of our teeth into old age or to prevent us getting toothache; it is also important for heart[7] and brain[8] health. So make sure dental care is one of your good habits for your overall health and wellbeing.

If you have a new habit you want to embed in your life, work out what will act as a reminder. Maybe you will need to set a reminder on your phone or pin up a note somewhere obvious, but if you can connect the new habit to something that is already a part of your routine, then give that a go. You may need to experiment with different reminders.

Some new habits are easier to stick to if you can do it with someone else. If you decide to go for a regular walk, arranging to go at a set time with a friend can make it much easier to stick to. The reminder is the commitment in the diary and the reward is twofold: the actual exercise plus the time with your friend, both of which are so important for wellbeing. Now have a think about something that you have wanted to add into your daily life for some time, but have struggled to find a way to make happen, and identify the possible *reminder*, *response* and *reward*.

Bad habits

I hope this has given you some ideas about forming new habits. But what about breaking bad habits? James Clear, author of *Atomic Habits*, suggests that bad habits are usually brought about by stress and boredom, and that if we want to break a bad habit, we need to replace it with a new one. If we go back to the reminder-response-reward cycle, first of all we need to try and remove as many of those reminders as possible. So if a biscuit habit is often triggered by spotting biscuits at the front of the cupboard, then you have a few possibilities for removing the reminder. You can move them to a more hidden place and put something healthier in their place instead, or you can stop buying them altogether. Keeping the temptation out of sight also works well if we want to cut down on phone use, as we are then less likely to keep checking our phones. In experiments it has been shown that people can concentrate better when their phones are not in view.[9] I often put mine away in a drawer if I am working on a concentrated piece of work. Having it visible on my desk is just too tempting.

Another way of getting rid of a bad habit is by replacing it with a good habit that brings about a similar type of reward. Going back to the biscuit example, if you are trying to give up biscuits then ask yourself what would give a similar type of reward. If you think you are craving something sweet, is there a healthier sweet snack that you could enjoy? I have found over the years that I have managed to replace my bad habit of eating lots of milk chocolate with a better habit of eating a small amount of dark chocolate (sometimes topped with nut butter and raisins – delicious!).

In order to make your bad habits harder and your good habits easier you need to change the reminders, and that might mean changing your environment. If you are trying to cut down on the amount of cake you eat, this might mean meeting friends for a walk rather than at a café – avoiding places that encourage your bad habits. Or to encourage a good habit of exercising, it might mean keeping exercise gear in a handy place rather than stowed away at the back of the garage. I use dumbbells as part of my morning fitness routine and they are kept in the bedroom, which is where I do my exercises. I know that if I had to go to another part of the house to find them every morning, I would never lift them up. They may not be the most beautiful interior decoration, but my physical health is more important. Now I would like you to take a few minutes to think about the following questions and see if they could help you to break a bad habit. Maybe, unlike me, you don't have any!

1. What bad habit (response) are you trying to give up if any?
2. What are the reminders (cues/triggers)?
3. What are the rewards?
4. Can you find a new habit (response) that gives you a similar reward?

Before we leave this milestone, I would like you to have a look at the list of small habits (on pages 187-188) that we might want to fit into our lives, and consider if they are already part of your life. For each one, consider if it is: already a habit for you; not something that you want or need in your life; or something you might like to add into your life. Then choose one new habit that you think would be beneficial to you, work out the reminder, response and reward, and then make a plan to experiment with getting that habit into your life. And remember to start small; be inspired by B J Fogg planning to floss just one tooth. In fact the smaller the habit, the better, as you are much more likely to stick with it. It is also important to think about the best place to fit your new habit into your day and to remember everyone is different. For example, some people prefer exercising in the morning, some people prefer after work or during lunch time. There is no right and wrong, only what is right for you (although it is best not to exercise late at night as it can interfere with sleep). If your desired new habit is to read more, when would it work best for you? Can you find a few minutes at lunchtime, or could you watch less TV and read for half an hour after dinner? What would suit you best?

It is also important to celebrate what you have achieved. Maybe you would be motivated by setting up a form of tracker (paper or electronic) to mark when you have achieved your habit for the day. You might then give yourself a small reward at the end of the month. Dr Chatterjee suggests popping a bean into a jar every time you do your new habit, maybe a coffee bean or something similar, and you will be able to see the progress you've made very visually. This serves as a powerful representation of your habit building. Or if you are starting up a new habit with another member of your family, you might like to set up a wall chart you can both add to. It is important to think realistically about what you know would motivate you. What might be motivating for one person might be irritating or a chore for someone else.

If you have taken the advice in this milestone seriously, then a new habit will not feel overwhelming and it will be just a small thing that you change in your life, but if you stick with it you will start to notice that it makes a big difference.

Below is a list of some habits – you may already do most of them, but are there any that you don't do that would be beneficial to add into your life on a regular basis?

1. Getting up and going to bed at a regular time each day
2. Making your bed
3. Brushing and flossing your teeth
4. Leaving for work on time
5. Carrying out strength exercises – push-ups, squats, lunges, dumbbells
6. Carrying out exercises for balance
7. Carrying out exercises for flexibility
8. Getting about 30 minutes of moderate exercise most days
9. Moving regularly during the day – using the stairs, etc.
10. Doing pelvic floor exercises
11. Attending health screening appointments such as dental check-ups, eye tests, hearing tests, cancer checks (not frequent but important)
12. Having a regular eating pattern
13. Eating in a set time window – time-restricted eating
14. Eating a wide variety of healthy food
15. Eating a healthy breakfast
16. Eating a healthy lunch
17. Eating a healthy dinner
18. Eating at least five portions of vegetables/fruit each day
19. Adding an extra portion of vegetables to each meal
20. Planning meals for the week
21. Eating fermented foods

22. Not eating in the two hours before bedtime
23. Staying hydrated by drinking enough fluids
24. Not drinking more than 14 units of alcohol a week
25. Having at least three alcohol-free days a week
26. Not watching excess TV/internet
27. Having quiet times e.g. – meditation, mindfulness, yoga
28. Establishing a short breathing practice
29. Talking to family and friends
30. Having a laugh
31. Helping neighbours or in your community
32. Living mainly in the present, not in the past or the future
33. Having smartphone-free time
34. Praying
35. Being grateful for the good things in your life
36. Spending time outside in the fresh air
37. Gardening
38. Growing herbs
39. Having time outdoors in the morning
40. Budgeting
41. Saving and investing for the future
42. Learning new information or skills
43. Being creative
44. Doing crosswords or puzzles
45. Listening to or playing music
46. Keeping a journal
47. Doing small acts of kindness
48. Making greener choices
49. Reducing the use of single-use plastics
50. Doing anything else that lifts you up and is good for your long-term wellbeing.

7:B – Support my willpower

The second milestone of Path 7 looks at ways to support your willpower so that you can increase the chances of making your planned changes stick. If willpower was an easy skill to turn on, we would never give up on a new year's resolution, fall off a healthy eating plan, give up on an exercise regime or stop a hobby, but everyone does at some time or another. So lacking in the willpower department is just another of the wonders of being a normal human being. Dr Kelly McGonigal, in her book *The Willpower Instinct*, provides lots of ideas and guidance on how to support your willpower. She also talks about 'won't power', as quite often we are trying not to do something – not to have that doughnut! And crucially we also need the ability to hold our long-term goal in our minds so that it can help us when we don't feel that we have very much willpower at all. In my case that long-term goal is to keep healthy, to fit into my clothes and not to have to buy a whole new wardrobe! So having a doughnut is a rare event.

Hopefully if you have only planned to make small changes you won't require much willpower to implement your new habits and to keep going with them, but we are all human. We often start off with great intentions which get lost in the busyness of our lives, so Kelly McGonigal's research provides some useful ideas for helping us to make change happen.

Routine

One of her tips is to automate the good habit, just as described in the previous milestone. Add the new habit on to an already established practice. Make it part of your routine. Routine is such a powerful way to establish good habits as it requires less thought and there is less likelihood of ducking out. For example, having a set bedtime routine of 10.30pm means you are very likely to get sufficient sleep every day rather than if your bedtime is erratic. Having a food plan means you are more likely to have healthy meals than if you only think about your food choices once you are hungry. Routine helps to keep you in harmony with your body clock (your circadian rhythm), which is increasingly being shown to improve health outcomes such as weight control, heart health and even mood. There is some really interesting research being carried out on how the timing of various aspects of our lifestyle, such as eating, sleeping and exercise, impacts on our health; for more information you can follow the work of Dr Satchin Panda[10] on the circadian clock.

Long term goals

As I mentioned before, having our overall long-term goal clear in our minds is very important. For example, if you decided to set up a chart to record your progress, then at the top in big letters include the overall goal, the reason you are doing this daily habit, and keep that at the forefront of your thoughts to increase your motivation when the going gets tough, as we know it will. Making this something you do with others or as a family can be really motivating too.

Meditation

Another way that has been shown to support willpower is to meditate. Meditation was discussed in Path 6 as a way to reduce stress, and it has also been shown to improve our willpower, another good reason for making a short meditation practice part of our daily lives. (Which comes first, the meditation practice or the willpower? Sounds a bit like a chicken and egg situation to me!)

Breath

Another willpower-enhancing tip is to take a number of deep breaths. When you catch yourself about to head for the biscuit tin for the second time, sit and take some deep breaths, slow your breathing down, bring your focus to your breath and see if that helps just break the automatic response that you're about to engage in. Remember that our good habits and our bad habits are very automated.

Nature

Getting outside into nature for a few minutes has been shown to help willpower. If you're trying to break a bad habit, try to notice when you get the reminder (the cue or trigger), and see if you can get outside for a little while and break the habit.

Ten minutes

Another way to help your willpower is to resist that thing you don't want to do for 10 minutes. Using the biscuit example, if you are trying to break the habit of a second biscuit, then just tell yourself, 'If I still feel like another biscuit in 10 minutes, then I can have one,' and go and find something to do for those 10 minutes. This can be a way of breaking the habit cycle. I have another use for the 10-minute rule: if there is good habit I want to incorporate into my day, but I don't feel like doing it, then telling myself I will just do it for 10 minutes is another way of getting going with it. I have used that so many times when writing this book. I was often not in the mood for working on it but really wanted to achieve my long-term goal of actually getting it finished. I would say to myself, 'Just do 10 minutes – surely you can manage 10 minutes,' and so often I would do many minutes more, hours even! Of course there are some things that once you start you need to keep going until they are finished, such as cooking a meal. You don't want to chop onions and start to cook some vegetables and then just give up, but there are many things that this tip is helpful for. If your new habit is to go for a 30-minute walk each day but you are just not in the mood for whatever reason, why not decide to go for just 10 minutes and see how you feel after that? Walk for five minutes, turn around and walk back. It's much better than not going at all. I used to abandon a planned walk if it was raining, claiming to be someone who hates the rain, but in recent times, unless the rain is very heavy, I don't let it put me off – and I have discovered, to my surprise, that I rather enjoy walking or running in the rain. Now rain and wind together, that is a different matter!

Be kind to myself

What should we do on the days when we do give up on our plans? As mentioned in Path 6, being kind to yourself when you fail, which you will do some of the time, can actually be better for your willpower in the future than being hard on yourself. So if you have planned to exercise for five minutes every morning for five days a week and you only manage three days, don't be too hard on yourself. Recognise what you have done, remember to be your own best friend and start afresh.

Plan ahead

Another tip for supporting your willpower is to plan ahead to develop strategies for when you know temptation will strike or when you know you are likely to duck out of a commitment. These are called 'if-then strategies', so if x happens then I will do y. For exercise it might be if it is raining heavily then I will do a YouTube exercise video instead. Planning ahead and having contingency plans engages the prefrontal cortex of your brain, rather than mainly relying on your more primitive automatic responses, and this can be a good strategy for improving your willpower and embedding new habits.

Remove temptation

Removing temptation is another really good strategy for supporting your willpower, and this is most obvious when you are trying to stop doing something like eating unhealthy snacks, smoking, or drinking alcohol or fizzy drinks. Having quick and easy access to the item in question makes it so much harder to stick to your plans, so clear out the cupboards, get rid of the tempting items and go and buy some healthier alternatives. When it comes to giving up smoking (or what has become the alternative, vaping), you are much more likely to succeed with professional help. Most health services have smoking-cessation support from local pharmacists or health centres.

Get support

Finding a role model can be another away to support you to achieve your new goals. People are often more successful at losing weight if they join a slimming club, or they do more exercise if they join a group or buddy up with someone. Ask yourself who you know who already does the habit that you want to establish. Can you talk to them about what motivates them, what benefits they have found from their habit, and how they have stuck with it? They will be able to give you a much better idea of the longer-term benefits of this new habit too, and this can be motivating at the start when the benefits are less tangible.

Having someone to hold you accountable is another good way of getting a new habit established. You could link this with the previous suggestion by asking your role model to hold you accountable. Maybe you could report in weekly about your progress. Having written goals that you report to somebody else has been shown to be one of the most effective ways of making progress.[11] It's often known as having an 'accountability partner'. I am not too keen on that phrase, but having someone else to report to can definitely help. I have known it to work very successfully for my coaching clients when they are studying for an exam or completing a thesis, so have a think about whether this is something you could harness to support your willpower.

Focus on the positive

Focusing on what you can do, or what you already have, is also a good way to support your willpower. For example, if you are trying to give something up, focus on what you have replaced it with. Or maybe you say before every exercise session, 'I'm thankful for being able to do these exercises, for being strong enough, for being fit enough, for having enough mobility.' Sometimes if I'm not in the mood for a planned walk or run I think about Melanie Reid. She is a *Times* journalist who was paralysed in a horse-riding accident many years ago. I say to myself, 'Melanie would love to be able to go out for a run right now,' and I count my blessings, put my shoes on and get going.

Surf the urge

My final tip for supporting your willpower is what's known as 'surfing the urge.'[12] When you notice the reminder for your habit, it starts the habit cycle, so be curious about what you are feeling. Do you remember the expansion exercise in Path 6? Why not try that when you are lacking willpower or 'won't power'. Notice what you are feeling in your body or your mind. What's going on for you? Is it a thought that is driving you, or an emotion? Can you locate it and picture it? Be curious about it, then describe it as an object, breathe around it and see if you can sit with it for 10 minutes. Then choose an action that you know will help you reach your long-term goal.

That brings us to the end of *Path 7 – Develop positive habits*. It brings together much of the work we have done in the previous six paths and hopefully helps you to identify some of the small changes that will have a big impact in your life. But remember to start small; this book is not about making massive changes that you'll be keen on for a while and then you'll forget all about. Small things done regularly are far better than big things done once and forgotten. And above all, be kind to yourself. Just do your best, as that's all we can ask of ourselves, and don't forget to remember the long-term goal and enjoy the journey.

Liv's story

One of the most important parts of the *Positive Paths to Wellbeing* course for me was the need to get more positive habits into my life, especially in the areas of personal wellbeing, diet and exercise. I have a very busy job and family life and mostly had been putting other people's needs before my own. The course really made me rethink that. *Path 5 – Look after my body* and *Path 7 – Develop positive habits* really focused me on making some changes. I started to implement time restricted eating, eating only between 11am and 7pm, making healthier food choices and cutting out any highly processed foods. I feel so much better as a result: sharper mind, lower blood pressure, weight loss and no more heartburn. I also worked out the best time to fit some daily exercises into my life. First thing in the morning has worked really well for me and I have my short fitness routine done and dusted before I start the day, just as Marie described in the course. I now make sure I take care of my own wellbeing, as without that I can't take care of others. I have a precious family and my job involves caring for others too, so by taking care of my own wellbeing I can be there for them now and in the future.

Path 8
Continue learning for life

'Anyone who stops learning is old, whether at twenty or eighty.
Anyone who keeps learning stays young.' Henry Ford

8:A – Continue learning for work

I am sure you will have heard the expression 'every day is a school day'. So just think for a minute about something you learnt yesterday. Maybe a new fact or a new skill, or maybe you cooked a new recipe or learnt a new shortcut on the computer. Maybe when you were talking to someone, they said something you hadn't known before, or you saw something new on the TV. Learning new knowledge and skills is good for you, for your brain and also for your mental health. Learning something new can boost your confidence, keep you up to date in your field of work and ensure you are ready for new challenges. And being interested in new things is both stimulating and energising. So in order to continue to grow and develop we need to keep on learning. This doesn't necessarily need to be formal learning: we can learn so much from our life experiences if we are open to them and enthusiastic.

I would like you to take a short pause now and think about some of the new things you have learnt in the last year or two. Make a note of any benefits you have gained from what you learnt. There is a list of potential benefits below – you may well have thought of others too.

- Builds confidence
- Builds a sense of self-worth
- Helps us connect with others
- Fuels creativity
- Can be fun
- Can help us make better use of time
- Reveals new talents
- Improves employment skills
- Makes us more adaptable to change
- Can help us earn more money
- Provides a good role-model for children
- Counteracts boredom
- Supports our career
- Stimulates the brain
- Slows cognitive decline
- Can improve our memory
- Can make us more productive

Were you surprised at how much you have learnt recently? I have completed a number of certificates and learnt so many new IT skills in the last few years, and it has enriched my life immeasurably. I have also learnt skills that are more for my leisure time, which we will look at more in the next milestone.

BASK

When I worked in staff development, I often helped people to develop their skills for work through workshops and coaching. A simple acronym that I used to help people analyse what they needed to focus on was BASK, where behaviour = attitude + skills + knowledge. (BASK was taught to me many years ago on a training course and I have since used it with many groups.) If the staff member wasn't getting the results they wanted through their current behaviour, I encouraged them to look at which of these three areas they needed to develop. Did they have the knowledge and skills required but their attitude was holding them back? Maybe they were struggling to work harmoniously with colleagues or clients. This was not uncommon and never an easy one to fix! Encouraging them to learn more about the soft skills required in the workplace and to seek out a coach or mentor was a good place to start. This is particularly an issue for new entrants to the workplace, either because it can take time to learn what is required for a workplace or because the workplace has a particular culture that they have not experienced before. You may have memories of starting a new job and finding there were all sorts of unwritten 'rules' that everyone seemed to know but were completely alien to you. Picking up the workplace culture can be so much more difficult than acquiring the knowledge and skills for the job.

While young people may take some time to pick up the workplace etiquette and culture, at the other end of the age scale I came across people who were reluctant to learn anything new as they considered themselves too old to learn. Personally I think this is what makes you old, not the other way round. Yes, as we get older it can be harder to learn new things. We might take longer to pick up and memorise new information, but age is certainly not a barrier to new learning. Motivation is what makes a big difference between learners and non-learners at any age.

Moving on from the A (attitude) of BASK, what about the S of skill and the K of knowledge? If someone is struggling with some tasks at work, do they need to do some more study, such as learn about a new technique or theory? Maybe there is a course they could attend in person or online or some reading they could do? Or do they have the knowledge but need support and practice to turn it into a skill? Often a mentor and the opportunity to practise can be all that is needed. Sometimes the missing skill is what is known as a soft skill, which can be a bit less obvious.

Take a look at the soft skills below. What would you add to this list for your workplace?

- Good communication skills
- Ability to relate to and empathise with others
- Patience
- Reliability – turning up, delivering on promises
- Working efficiently
- Ability to prioritise
- Ability to trust others
- Good listening skills

- Ability to resolve conflicts
- Interested in the work and the people
- Good judgement
- Creative
- Critical thinker
- Flexible
- Persuasive
- Able to support and motivate
- Open-minded
- Diplomatic honesty
- Ability to problem solve
- Sense of humour
- Good manners
- Good hygiene!

Have a think about whether there is a behaviour you want to develop for your work. 'Behaviour' might seem a strange way to describe it, so you can substitute that with 'working practice' or 'way of working' if that makes more sense to you. Now think about what is preventing you from doing this behaviour. Is it attitude (or maybe a softer way of putting that is 'your approach') or your knowledge or your skills? Let me give you an example.

At the end of 2019 I decided that I wanted to change my *Positive Paths to Wellbeing* workshop (that I delivered in person) into an online course. The desired 'behaviour' was to produce videos of the workshop content. What was my attitude? I was very keen to learn, and I was prepared to put in the hard work, so it was looking good on the attitude front. What about knowledge? That was seriously lacking. I knew it was possible but that was about all, so I attended a Business Gateway workshop and used YouTube videos to add to my knowledge. Translating that knowledge into a skill took a lot more time, patience and practice, but I got there! As my business develops, I still need to learn new knowledge and skills on a regular basis, and I still frequently have to google to get answers to fill my knowledge gaps. But I love learning for work, so every time I solve a 'puzzle' I get such a buzz. That is not to say that on some days, and for some areas where I lack the necessary knowledge, my attitude is less than enthusiastic. Marketing and advertising are definitely areas that I have a bit of a block about.

Do take a moment to pause now and think about something that you would like to be able to do for work (that could be paid or unpaid, such as running a home and family), and use BASK to analyse what you need to do to move forward.

Ways of learning

Now that we have considered what you have learnt in recent times and the three main components of behaviour – attitude, skills and knowledge – I want you to think about all of the different ways of learning. So take a few moments to think about how you have gained, or could gain, new attitudes, skills and knowledge.

There are so many ways to learn in addition to the obvious formal options such as qualifications. I have listed some below and I am sure you can think of more. Which of these methods of learning is the most useful for your line of work?

- Reading
- Courses – in person and online
- Formal qualifications
- Experimenting
- Shadowing a colleague
- Finding a mentor
- Reflective writing
- Skills practice
- Trial and learn
- Coaching
- On-the-job training
- Instructional videos
- TED talks
- Audio/podcasts

Career development

What if you don't feel your current working situation is right for you? Maybe you feel that you were pushed down a particular career path by family expectations or school-teachers, or because you just did not know what you wanted to do when you left school and had to pick something, anything. If that sounds like you, remember that there are experts in career development who can help you if you feel you are needing a change of direction. I have had a number of significant changes during my working life and I truly believe that it is possible to change direction. You can use the skills you have, and your capacity and enthusiasm to develop new skills, to help you grow, develop and change throughout your working life. In this way, work stays fresh, relevant, motivating and rewarding for the rest of your life. I certainly have no plans to put my feet up and retire as long as I can keep helping people live calmer, happier, healthier lives. Studies have shown that retiring early can speed up cognitive decline,[1] so whilst we might moan about work on a regular basis, the mental stimulation and the social connection is very good for us. The best thing is to find a job we enjoy, and then when the time is right, move on to an active and stimulating retirement.

Now take a few minutes to answer the questions below and think about what your future working life might hold for you.

1. How are you keeping up to date in your career?
2. How would you like your career to evolve in the future?
3. Do you need some support to plan for your future career?

Over the years I have worked with a number of people who have not enjoyed their job, but family circumstances understandably made them reluctant to take a risk on a new career. I encouraged them to have a think about BASK. Was there one element that needed some focus? Were their knowledge and skills up to date? Was there anything they could do to change their attitude to the work? I am reminded of the old proverb of two stonemasons working on the construction of a cathedral that would not be completed until long after their deaths. When asked what they were doing, one replied, 'I am chiselling stone,' and the other stonemason replied, 'I am building a cathedral to the glory of God and mankind.' Same job, different attitude. I wonder who enjoyed their job more?

8:B – Continue learning for leisure

One thing that has been a constant throughout my life is the need for some sort of craft or creative hobby. From a young age I have loved making things, and I know that if I don't make something every now and again, I start to feel as though something isn't right. When I analyse why I might not be feeling quite 'me' and I am a bit lower on the Scale of Wellbeing, I recognise that my creative outlet has been shut down for a while.

Creativity comes in many forms. Whether it is gardening, sewing, cooking, playing music or making videos, there are countless ways to be creative. The *Oxford English Dictionary's* definition of the word creativity is 'the use of skill and imagination to produce something new'. And creativity is increasingly seen to be essential to a person's wellbeing.[2]

The psychologist Mihaly Csikszentmihalyi was famous for his studies on happiness.[3] He identified that the best times in our lives are when we are absorbed in something that is achievable but challenging. He calls this 'flow', (which was introduced in *6:B — Live in the moment*), and many creative or leisure tasks can really absorb us and bring us into 'flow', and of course this can apply to a satisfying work task too. So consider when you were last in 'flow', when you were fully absorbed in the task and you were not aware of the passage of time – maybe it speeded up or slowed down. Another expression we can use for this feeling is 'being in the zone'.

Of course, leisure time is not all about creativity. It is also about physical activity such as sport and exercise or maybe soaking up some culture or enjoying your favourite TV programme. It might be about spending time with family and friends. Basically it is what you spend your time doing when work and chores are done. And there are real benefits to leisure time. It has been shown to lower heart rates, reduce stress and promote a better mood.[4] Why not pause your reading for a few minutes and make a list of the activities you do in your leisure time and then make a note about the benefits they bring to your life?

Not all of the activities that take up your leisure time will require much learning. Watching the TV, going for a walk and having fun with friends are all things we don't need any extra training for. But there are other leisure activities that we can improve on and that we can enjoy learning more about. Taking music lessons, attending an evening class, watching YouTube videos to learn something for your hobby, going to an art club to learn from more experienced people, and having swimming lessons are just some examples of how you can learn for your leisure time.

Trial and learn

Improving through trial and error, such as by attempting more difficult puzzles, is another way of learning. I prefer to think of it as 'trial and learn' rather than 'trial and error'. If we think critically about what we are doing, then we most certainly will be learning from any 'errors' we make – so don't think of them as errors, but ways of learning. Many business development leaders emphasise the need to learn from our mistakes. When we push ourselves out of our comfort zone, we inevitably will make mistakes. But what is the alternative – to stay still and to hold ourselves back?

Comfort zone

I can't remember where I heard the following analogy, so apologies for not being able to name the person who inspired me with this. We can think of our comfort zone as a hula hoop which we are standing in. This is a hula hoop made of plastic, the sort that I tried unsuccessfully as a child to spin around my waist. So the comfort zone hula hoop is just big enough for us to stand in. When we think about doing something challenging, something outside our comfort zone, we don't want to try something a long way outside of this hoop; but we can try something just a little way out, and we should. Take a small step that still feels like a challenge, but an achievable one. In this way we increase the size of our hoop. If we aim for too big a step, we may well fail, and this reduces the likelihood of us trying again. It goes back to my philosophy that small, consistent steps over time build into big steps in the end.

Look at the list below of ways of learning for leisure and see what would help you to take a small step out of your comfort zone.

- Community/evening classes
- Creative clubs and groups
- Book clubs
- Sports groups
- Exercise classes
- Dance classes
- YouTube videos
- College courses
- Qualifications/exams
- Reading

- Trial and learn
- Mentor/expert input
- Private lessons
- TED talks

- Online courses
- Workshops
- Instruction guides
- Practice

Finding time

What about finding the time for leisure activities? Your current life circumstances might not allow much time for leisure. Maybe you have a busy work life and a busy home life, or you have young children (and I remember how demanding and exhausting that time was). Or maybe on top of work and a family you have elderly relatives or a child with additional support needs. How can you find time for any leisure? I think this links us all the way to *Path 1 – Clarify what is important to me*. Maybe there are some things that are taking time in our lives that are less important. When I started my personal development journey and really delved deep into where I was putting my time, I realised I worried too much about housework and not enough about time with my children, so that was a bit of an eye opener. And I also knew that at that stage of my life, with young children, I couldn't have much leisure time on my own, so I looked at how best to have leisure time with my children. One thing we did was to sit as a family each evening whilst I read a chapter of Harry Potter to them. It actually satisfied my need for reading and was a lovely ritual that ended the day peacefully. So sometimes we need to get creative with how to be creative!

I want to emphasise again that no one is perfect. Be realistic and don't be a perfectionist. At busy stages of your life, find the creative outlet that gives you the most benefit in the least amount of time and prioritise that. For me that is reading. The opportunity to escape to another world with fiction or to keep learning by listening to a non-fiction audio book is one of the best uses of my leisure time. I also listen to audio books and podcasts whilst I am driving. I once saw that described as the 'university of the car' and that can be applied to other journeys too. Just make sure it does not compromise your safety in any way. Look for ways to use any spare time you have, to move you up the wellbeing scale. And remember it will be different for you – I have just given you my example here to illustrate the point.

Now spend some time thinking about which creative outlet really delivers the best rewards for you, and where it can fit into your life.

8:C – Continue learning for the future

This is the part where we wrap up the learning and take a look at how you can continue to use the life skills that have been covered throughout the book. My aim when I wrote the *Positive Paths to Wellbeing* course, which then became this book, was to develop a framework to sum up the life skills that I was lucky enough to learn during my working life. I hope that when you find yourself with a problem of some sort you can ask yourself which path or milestone would help you think more deeply about it, and help you find a way forward.

If, for example, the issue you are having is on physical health, you can revisit *Path 5 – Look after my body* and decide what you would like to try and change. If your issue is with a relationship with a friend, family member or work colleague, you can revisit the relationship building exercise from *Path 3 – Nurture my relationships* and also *Path 4 – Improve communication*. This might help you gently initiate a conversation in order to find a way to improve your relationship.

What if you are finding yourself stressed and anxious? You can revisit the Wheel of Wellbeing from Path 1 to analyse if there is a particular area of your life you need to focus on. You can also revisit *Path 6 – Look after my mind*, and you might find you need to look after your body too.

What if you are having difficult relationships with children? You can teach them about the relationship house (Path 3) and plan together how you can look after your 'house', not knock it down. Or maybe you plan together some fun leisure time that would benefit everyone (Path 8). Or you can work through the six-step conflict-resolution process from Path 4, teaching them the steps along the way.

What if you are being too hard on yourself and lacking in confidence? Maybe revisiting Path 6 will help you to be kinder to yourself. Or maybe developing small, positive habits from Path 7 will increase your self-esteem as you make commitments and achieve them. Or maybe Path 8 inspires you to learn more about self-confidence and how to boost it.

And what if you are run ragged with just too much to do? Maybe you can revisit Path 1 and work out what is important to you, then Path 2 to work out how to fit these things into your life. And maybe Path 7 can help you find small steps to move in the direction you want to go, whilst still being kind to yourself (Path 6) when you inevitably fall short of the ideal.

In all of these problems one of the first things to consider, and for me the most important concept of all, is the circle of control. What is in your direct control? There really is no point wasting energy on things we don't have any control over. Now I know that is easier said than done, but remember the only person you have direct control over is yourself, and even then there are parts of our thoughts and feelings we don't have direct, conscious control over. So can we really expect to have control over someone else? Although, our actions undoubtedly do influence others, for better or worse.

Take a few minutes to think of a problem that could do with some thought, then look at the *Positive Paths to Wellbeing* infographic (page 9) and work out what tools and concepts you could use to start you along the path to a solution. Sometimes there will not be any obvious, neat solution, and you still won't know what to do for the best. Life can be very complicated. You might find that speaking to a counsellor, coach or mentor can help you to think more deeply. And, importantly, keep being kind to yourself as you work out a way forward. Life can be messy, and no one has all the answers, so just keep doing your best. No one has had your background; no one has had your experiences. I heard Dr Chatterjee say that he always tries to accept people as they are, and to remember that if he had exactly the same life experiences as them, he would probably be in the same situation as them, so he does not judge. I think that is such a lovely attitude to have and one that I try to adopt too.

As we approach the end of the book, I want to remind you of something I introduced back in the third milestone of Path 1 (*1:C Plan the future*). I said we would come back to it at the end – well, I haven't forgotten! We are going to have a little look into the future. I want you to sit comfortably and take a few slow breaths, breathing in for 4 and out for 6. Imagine your journey over the next six months. I want you to imagine what may have changed for you, not lottery wins or things outside your control but changes that you can bring about by your focus and your actions.

- What small steps will you be taking every day along the journey?
- What new things will you be discovering?
- Who will you be connecting with?
- What will be supporting you along the way, not to a final goal but to this waypoint on your journey through life?
- Who are the key people on your journey?
- How are you feeling in mind and body?
- What is inspiring you and lifting you up the Scale of Wellbeing?

Hold that image in your mind and spend a few minutes filling out the vision exercise below.

My name is:

It is (date):

I have had a _____ six months and here are the reasons why:

I don't want you to pass over this exercise. Remember you haven't been to Peru if you have only read the guidebook! (Why do I always picture Paddington Bear when I think of that?) Spend a good few minutes thinking this through and writing it down. It can be very detailed actions or high-level values and philosophy, whatever is right for you. Maybe a mixture of both. I did this exercise when I was training as a coach and found it really helped me to focus on passing my course and to achieve my coaching qualification. I even predicted the date I would receive my certificate, which was rather spooky! It also inspired me to make my dream of having my own business a reality, so you never know what it might inspire you to do. Once you have written your vision you can come back to it again and again and review it, add to it, change it. It is not meant to be set in stone, but rather a motivational tool for increasing the likelihood of making changes. You could put it somewhere prominent, somewhere you will see it regularly, or tuck it away out of sight of anyone else. As always, do what is right for you. I hope you can use it to guide you for the next six months and beyond.

So that is us at the end of the eight paths. I can't thank you enough for reading my book and I hope it has inspired you to take positive steps to support your wellbeing.

Lynda's story

I came across the *Positive Paths to Wellbeing* course when I was looking for a programme for my team. It was during the time when we were starting to come out of the pandemic, and the online nature of the programme worked well for us as we were all working in different places, with some staff working from home and feeling a bit isolated. Lifelong learning is really important to me, and although all of the pathways felt relevant for us as a team, *Path 8* –really resonated with me. This programme was an opportunity to continue learning about wellbeing, and also for us to connect as a team. Most people completed the programme, and everyone gained different things from it, depending on their individual circumstances. It really helped us as a team to reconnect as well as get to know each other better, and it helped us to move forward at this difficult time. After the programme finished, we were much more proactive about checking in with each other and making sure everyone was doing well, encouraging a culture of asking for support if needed. We wanted to keep a focus on wellbeing. It gave us permission to put aside the work agenda at agreed times and to focus on the human connection. Some staff members also took advantage of some coaching sessions, which they found very beneficial. Having a culture of looking after our own wellbeing as well as caring for the wellbeing of the whole team benefitted everyone, and helped foster relationships and build resilience.

Dear Reader,

Now that we have finished the eight paths, I hope this book has helped you in some small way. Sometimes I find 'self-help' or 'personal development' books a bit too unrealistic and seem to be expecting us to change into perfectly programmed robots rather than recognising that we are actual human beings. I really hope that *Positive Paths to Wellbeing* does not feel that way. I want you to be kind to yourself, and if you make one or two small changes, or even none at all, that is just fine. It is entirely up to you. One thing I know for sure is that no human life is perfect. Most of us are doing our best given our genetics, the life experiences that have shaped us and the environment we are in. So if we can keep that in mind and know that most others are doing the same, maybe we can be kinder to ourselves and to those we meet along this journey in life.

I have absolutely loved writing this book and I am so glad that you have joined me on this journey. Please do keep in touch by signing up for my newsletter at my website www.mariepaterson.com, where you can also find out more about my wellbeing coaching, training and team programmes. Thank you so much for reading my book, and keep following your own positive paths.

With warmest wishes

Marie

Resources

The resources listed here are to provide ideas for further study. Including them here does not mean I agree with everything they contain, but they are interesting resources for further information on wellbeing. Weblinks accessed November 2023.

Introduction

Covey SR, 1989. *The 7 Habits of Highly Effective People*. New York: Simon & Schuster.

Frankl VE, 2004. *Man's Search for Meaning.* London: Rider.

Path 2 – Take personal responsibility

Allen D, 2001. *Getting Things Done*. London: Piatkus.

Canfield J, 2005. *The Success Principles.* New York: Harper Collins.

Covey S, 1999. *The 7 Habits of Highly Effective Teenagers.* London: Simon & Schuster.

Harris R, 2021. *The Happiness Trap.* 2nd edition. London: Robinson.

Kondo M, 2014. *The Life-Changing Magic of Tidying.* London: Vermillion.

Tracy B, 2013. *Eat that Frog*. London: Yellow Kite.

Path 3 – Nurture my relationships

Covey SR, *The 7 Habits of Highly Effective Families.* Revised edition. 2022. New York: Golden Press.

Perel E, 2007. *Mating in captivity*. London: Hodder & Stoughton

Perry P, 2020. *The book you wish your parents had read*. London: Penguin Life.

Perry P, 2023. *The Book You Want Everyone You Love* To Read *(and maybe a few you don't)*. London: Cornerstone Press.

Path 4 – Improve communication

Fisher R & Ury W, 1992. *Getting to Yes.* 2nd edition. London: Random House.

Path 5 – Look after my body

Aujla R, 2017. *The Doctor's Kitchen*. London: Thorsons.

Carr A, 2015. Allen Carr's *Easy Way to Stop Smoking*. London: Penguin.

Chatterjee R, 2019. *Feel Better in 5*. London: Penguin Life.

Chatterjee R, 2020. *Feel Great, Lose Weight*. London: Penguin Life.

Dreyer D, 2004. *Chi Running*. New York: Simon & Schuster.

Fung J & Moore J, 2016. *The Complete Guide to Fasting*. Las Vegas: Victory Belt.

Galloway J, 2016. *The Run Walk Run Method*. UK: Meyer and Meyer Sport.

Gregory A, 2020. *Nodding Off*. London: Bloomsbury Sigma.

Hameed S, 2022. *The Full Diet*. London: Michael Joseph.

Jacka F, 2019. *Brain Changer*. London: Yellow Kite.

Jenkinson A, 2021. *Why We Eat Too Much*. London: Penguin Life.

Mosley M, 2020. *Fast Asleep*. London: Short Books.

Mosley M & Spencer M, 2014. *The Fast Diet*. London: Short Books.

Mosley M, 2013. *Fast Exercise*. London: Short Books.

Nestor J, 2021. *Breath*. London: Penguin Life.

Oliver J. 2023. *5 Ingredients Mediterranean*. London: Michael Joseph.

Palmer C, 2022. *Brain Energy*. Dallas: Benbella Books.

Pelz M, 2022. *Fast Like a Girl*. London: Hay House.

Pinnock D, 2019. *Eat Shop Save: 8 Weeks to Better Health*. London: Hamlyn.

Ramage A & Fairbairns R, 2017. *The 28 Day Alcohol-Free Challenge*. London: Bluebird.

Rossi M, 2019. *Eat Yourself Healthy*. London: Penguin Life.

Spector T, 2015. *The Diet Myth*. London: Weidenfeld & Nicolson.

Stephens G. *Fast, Feast, Repeat*. New York: St Martin's Griffin.

Walker M, 2017. *Why We Sleep*. London: Penguin Books.

Wheatley-McGrain C, 2022. *Calm Your Gut*. London: Hay House.

Wicks J, *Feel Good Food*. London: HQ.

Parkrun. https://www.parkrun.org.uk/

Sleepio. Cognitive behaviour therapy for insomnia. https://www.sleepio.com/

Sleepstation. https://www.sleepstation.org.uk/

The Insomnia Clinic. https://www.theinsomniaclinic.co.uk/

Path 6 – Look after my mind

Chatterjee R, 2022. *Happy Mind, Happy Life*. London: Penguin Life.

Harris R, 2021. *The Happiness Trap*. 2nd edition. London: Robinson.

Huebener D, 2006. *What To Do When You Worry Too Much*.
    Washington DC: Magination Press. (Children's book.)

Lalli G, 2021. *How to Empty Your Stress Bucket*. UK: Tonic Titles.

Smith J. 2022. *Why Has Nobody Told Me This Before?* London: Michael
    Joseph.

Williams M & Penman D, 2011. *Mindfulness*. London: Piatkus.

Calm. Sleep and stress reduction app. https://www.calm.com/

Headspace. Meditation app. https://www.headspace.com/

Insight Timer. For guided meditations. https://insighttimer.com/

Mind. https://www.mind.org.uk/

NHS Better Health: Every Mind Matters. https://www.nhs.uk/every-
    mind-matters/

Samaritans. https://www.samaritans.org/

Sane. https://www.sane.org.uk/

Path 7 – Develop positive habits

Chatterjee R, 2019. *Feel Better in 5*. London: Penguin Life.

Clear J, 2018. *Atomic Habits.* London: Random House Business.

Fogg BJ, 2020. *Tiny Habits.* London: Virgin Books.

McGonigal K, 2013. *The Willpower Instinct*. New York: Avery.

Olson J, 201. *The Slight Edge*. 3rd edition. Austin: Greenleaf.

Panda S, 2018. *The Circadian Code.* London: Vermillion.

Other resources

Bartlett S, 2023. *The Diary of a CEO: The 33 Laws of Business & Life*.
    London: Penguin.

McCall D & Potter N. 2022. *Menopausing.* London: HQ.

Newson L, 2023. *The Definitive Guide to the Perimenopause and
    Menopause*. London: Yellow Kite.

Panja A, 2023. *The Health Fix*. London: Kyle Books.

References

Weblinks accessed November 2023.

Introduction

1. Covey SR, 2017. Foreword to Pattakos A. *Prisoners of our Thoughts.* https://www.viktorfrankl.org/assets/pdf/Covey_Intro_to_Pattakos _Prisoners.pdf

Path 2 – Take personal responsibility

1. Šimić G, et al. Understanding emotions: Origins and roles of the amygdala. *Biomolecules*. 2021;11(6):823.
2. Kassel G. This is how your brain develops in your teenage years. 2023. https://www.healthline.com/health/teen-brain-development
3. Berenholtz SM. Checklist cuts lethal ventilator-associated lung infections. 2011. https://www.hopkinsmedicine.org/news/media/releases/ checklist_cuts_lethal_ventilator_associated_lung_infections
4. Forest app. https://www.forestapp.cc/
5. Allen S. The science of gratitude. 2018. https://ggsc.berkeley.edu/ images/uploads/GGSC-JTF_White_Paper-Gratitude-FINAL.pdf
6. Moralis S & Dinan S. The myth of multitasking. 2022. https://www.psychologytoday.com/gb/blog/the-therapeutic-perspective/202202/the-myth-multitasking
7. Bindamnan A. Trying to multitask well? Just focus on one thing. 2023. https://www.psychologytoday.com/intl/blog/zero-generation-students/202303/trying-to-multitask-well-just-focus-on-one-thing

Path 3 – Nurture my relationships

1. Women's Aid. https://www.womensaid.org.uk/ Relate. https://www.relate.org.uk/get-help/emotional-abuse NHS. https://www.nhs.uk/live-well/getting-help-for-domestic-violence

Path 5 – Look after my body

1. Monteiro C, et al. Ultra-processed foods: what they are and how to identify them. *Public Health Nutrition*. 2019;22(5):936–941.

2. Vegan Society. https://www.vegansociety.com/

3. Newman T. Are seed oils bad for you? 2022. https://zoe.com/learn/are-seed-oils-bad-for-you

4. Zumpano J. Seed oils: Are they actually toxic? 2023. https://health.clevelandclinic.org/seed-oils-are-they-actually-toxic/

5. Manian C. What's the deal with seed oils – are they really so bad for you? 2023. https://www.realsimple.com/are-seed-oils-bad-for-you-6835267

6. Teicholz N. A short history of saturated fat: the making and unmaking of a scientific consensus. *Current Opinion in Endocrinology, Diabetes, and Obesity*. 2023;30(1):65–71.

7. Harvard Health Publishing. The truth about fats: the good, the bad, and the in-between. 2022. https://www.health.harvard.edu/staying-healthy/the-truth-about-fats-bad-and-good

8. Temple NJ. Fat, sugar, whole grains and heart disease: 50 years of confusion. *Nutrients*. 2018;10(1):39.

9. Cancer Research UK. Does eating processed and red meat cause cancer? 2023. https://www.cancerresearchuk.org/about-cancer/causes-of-cancer/diet-and-cancer/does-eating-processed-and-red-meat-cause-cancer

10. NHS. Red meat and the risk of bowel cancer. 2021. https://www.nhs.uk/live-well/eat-well/food-guidelines-and-food-labels/red-meat-and-the-risk-of-bowel-cancer/

11. NHS. Salt in your diet. 2023. https://www.nhs.uk/live-well/eat-well/food-types/salt-in-your-diet/

12. Action on salt. Salt and health factsheets. 2023. https://www.actiononsalt.org.uk/salthealth/factsheets/

13. Feel better, live more podcast. The new science of eating well with Professor Tim Spector. 2023. https://drchatterjee.com/the-new-science-of-eating-well-with-professor-tim-spector/

14. Taylor RS, et al. Reduced dietary salt for the prevention of cardiovascular disease: a meta-analysis of randomised controlled

trials (Cochrane review). *American Journal of Hypertension*. 2011;24(8):843–853.

15. He FJ, et al. Salt reduction to prevent hypertension and cardiovascular disease: JACC state-of-the-art review. Journal of the American College of Cardiology. 2020;75(6):632-647.

16. Diabetes UK. Low-carb diet and meal plan. 2023. https://www.diabetes.org.uk/guide-to-diabetes/enjoy-food/eating-with-diabetes/meal-plans/low-carb

17. Buettner D, 2012. *The Blue Zones*. Washington, DC: National Geographic.

18. Diabetes UK. Diabetes risk factors. 2023. https://www.diabetes.org.uk/diabetes-the-basics/types-of-diabetes/type-2/diabetes-risk-factors

19. NHS. Obesity. 2023. https://www.nhs.uk/conditions/obesity/

20. LeWine HE. Distracted eating may lead to weight gain. 2013. Harvard Health Publishing. https://www.health.harvard.edu/blog/distracted-eating-may-add-to-weight-gain-201303296037

21. Ajmera R. Eight health benefits of fasting, backed by science. 2023. https://www.healthline.com/nutrition/fasting-benefits#inflammation

22. Vetter C. Can intermittent fasting improve your gut health? 2023. https://zoe.com/learn/intermittent-fasting-gut-health

23. Anander L. Why is my blood sugar high in the morning? 2021. https://www.webmd.com/diabetes/morning-high-blood-sugar-levels

24. Mosley M, 2014. *The Fast Diet*. London: Short Books.

25. World Health Organisation. Aspartame hazard and risk assessment results released. 2023. https://www.who.int/news/item/14-07-2023-aspartame-hazard-and-risk-assessment-results-released

26. Brincat C. Do no-calorie artificial sweeteners have any effect on gut health and metabolism? 2022. https://www.medicalnewstoday.com/articles/do-no-calorie-artificial-sweeteners-have-any-effect-on-gut-health-or-metabolism

27. WebMD. What is too much water intake? 2023.
    https://www.webmd.com/diet/what-is-too-much-water-intake

28. Wikipedia. List of marathon fatalities. 2023.
    https://en.wikipedia.org/wiki/List_of_marathon_fatalities

29. Saner E. Have we had our fill of water? 2011. https://www.the
    guardian.com/society/2011/jul/22/had-our-fill-of-water

30. NHS Better Health. Drink less. 2023. https://www.nhs.uk/better-
    health/drink-less/

31. Alcoholics Anonymous. https://www.alcoholics-
    anonymous.org.uk/
    Al-Anon Family Groups UK & Eire. For families affected by
    alcohol. https://al-anonuk.org.uk/
    One Year No Beer. https://www.oneyearnobeer.com/
    Sober Sistas. https://sobersistas.co.uk/
    NHS. Alcohol support. https://www.nhs.uk/live-well/alcohol-
    advice/alcohol-support/
    NHS. Drug addiction support. https://www.nhs.uk/live-
    well/addiction-support/drug-addiction-getting-help/

32. NHS. Vitamin D. 2020. https://www.nhs.uk/conditions/vitamins-
    and-minerals/vitamin-d/

33. The Vegan Society. What every vegan should know about
    vitamin B12. 2023. https://www.vegansociety.com/
    resources/nutrition-and-health/nutrients/vitamin-b12/what-every-
    vegan-should-know-about-vitamin-b12

34. Scientific American. Dirt poor: Have fruits and vegetables
    become less nutritious? 2011. https://www.scientific
    american.com/article/soil-depletion-and-nutrition-loss/

35. Baker LD, et al. Effects of cocoa extract and a multivitamin on
    cognitive function: A randomised clinical trial. *Alzheimer's and
    Dementia*. 2023;19(4):1308–1309.

36. Move it or lose it. https://www.moveitorloseit.co.uk/

37. Downey A. Can you do too much exercise? 2020.
    https://patient.info/news-and-features/is-too-much-exercise-bad-
    for-you

38. Whiteman H. Now too much standing is bad for us, says study. 2018. https://www.medicalnewstoday.com/articles/321084

39. UK Chief Medical Officers' Physical Activity Guidelines. 2019. https://assets.publishing.service.gov.uk/media/5d839543ed915d5 2428dc134/uk-chief-medical-officers-physical-activity-guidelines.pdf

40. Denworth L. You don't really need 10,000 daily steps to be healthy. 2023. https://www.scientificamerican.com/article/you-dont-really-need-10-000-daily-steps-to-stay-healthy/

41. Adamakis M. 7 minute workout: High intensity circuit training. Technical report. 2018. https://www.researchgate.net/publication /327253837_7_minute_workout_High_intensity_circuit_training

42. Springer B, et al. Normative values for the unipedal stance test with eyes open and closed. *Journal of Geriatric Physical Therapy*. 2007;30(1):8–15.

43. World Health Organization. Falls. 2021. https://www.who.int/news-room/fact-sheets/detail/falls

44. Volpi E, et al. Muscle tissue changes with aging. *Current Opinion in Clinical Nutrition and Metabolic Care*. 2004;7(4):405–410.

45. NHS. Fitness Studio exercise videos. https://www.nhs.uk/conditions/nhs-fitness-studio/

46. Chaput J-P, et al. Sleeping hours: what is the ideal number and how does age impact this? *Nature and Science of Sleep*. 2018;10:421–430.

47. Corliss J. Addressing poor sleep may help heart health. 2022. https://www.health.harvard.edu/blog/struggling-to-sleep-your-heart-may-pay-the-price-202203092701

48. Bryant E. Lack of sleep in middle age may increase dementia risk. 2021. https://www.nih.gov/news-events/nih-research-matters/lack-sleep-middle-age-may-increase-dementia-risk

49. Randall DK. Insomnia: relax and stop worrying about lack of sleep. 2012. https://www.theguardian.com/ lifeandstyle/2012/sep/22/dreamland-insomnia-sleep-cbt-drugs

50. Wikipedia. Sleep inertia. 2023. https://en.wikipedia.org/wiki/Sleep_inertia

51. Harvard Health Publishing. Blue light has a dark side. 2020. https://www.health.harvard.edu/staying-healthy/blue-light-has-a-dark-side

52. University of Manchester. Blue light may not be as disruptive to our sleep patterns as originally thought. 2019. https://www.sciencedaily.com/releases/2019/12/191216173654.htm

53. Maurer LF, et al. The clinical effects of sleep restriction therapy for insomnia: A meta-analysis of randomised controlled trials. *Sleep Medicine Reviews*. 2021;58:101493.

54. Jennings KA. Does magnesium help you sleep better? 2023. https://www.healthline.com/nutrition/magnesium-and-sleep

55. Van de Walle G & West H. Magnesium supplements: All you need to know. 2023. https://www.healthline.com/nutrition/magnesium-supplements

56. NICE. What are the diagnostic criteria for insomnia? 2022. https://cks.nice.org.uk/topics/insomnia/diagnosis/clinical-features/

57. Mind. Sleeping pills and minor tranquillisers. 2021. https://www.mind.org.uk/information-support/drugs-and-treatments/sleeping-pills-and-minor-tranquillisers/about-sleeping-pills-and-minor-tranquillisers/

58. Balban MY, et al. Brief structured respiration practices enhance mood and reduce physiological arousal. *Cell Reports Medicine*. 2023;4(1);100895.

59. Huberman A. Breathing techniques to reduce stress and anxiety. 2021. https://www.youtube.com/watch?v=kSZKIupBUuc

60. Gillihan SJ. Frustrated you can't sleep? Try staying awake instead. 2018. https://www.psychologytoday.com/gb/blog/think-act-be/201804/frustrated-you-cant-sleep-try-staying-awake-instead

61. Pauwaert K, et al. Nocturia through the menopausal transition and beyond: A narrative review. *International Urogynecology Journal*. 2021;32(5):1097–1106.

62. NHS Inform. Benign prostate enlargement. 2023. https://www.nhsinform.scot/illnesses-and-conditions/kidneys-

bladder-and-prostate/benign-prostate-enlargement/#symptoms-of-benign-prostate-enlargement

63. Muench A, et al. We know CBT-I works, now what? *Faculty Reviews*. 2022;11:4.

Path 6 – Look after my mind

1. Festinger L. A theory of social comparison processes. *Human Relations*. 1954;7(2):117–140.

2. Self-compassion: Dr Kristin Neff. https://self-compassion.org/

3. Zollars I, et al. Effects of mindfulness meditation on mindfulness, mental well-being, and perceived stress. *Currents in Pharmacy Teaching and Learning.* 2019;11(10):1022–1028.

4. Whitton T, et al. How a mindfulness intervention can affect patients' mental wellbeing. *Nursing Times* [online]; 2019;115(7):48–51.

5. NICE. Depression in adults: treatment and management. 2022. https://www.nice.org.uk/guidance/ng222

6. Williams M & Penman D. 2011. *Mindfulness*. London: Piatkus. Online course - https://www.bemindfulonline.com/

7. Hofmann SG, et al. The effect of mindfulness-based therapy on anxiety and depression: A meta-analytic review. *Journal of Consulting and Clinical Psychology*. 2010;78(2):169–183.

8. Allen S. The science of gratitude. 2018. https://ggsc.berkeley.edu/images/uploads/GGSC-JTF_White_Paper-Gratitude-FINAL.pdf

9. Naumann J, et al. Effects and feasibility of hyperthermic baths in comparison to exercise as add-on treatment to usual care in depression: A randomised, controlled pilot study. *BMC Psychiatry*. 2020;20:536.

10. Dreisoerner A, et al. Self-soothing touch and being hugged reduce cortisol responses to stress: A randomised controlled trial on stress, physical touch, and social identity. *Comprehensive Psychoneuroendocrinology*. 2021;8:100091.

Path 7 – Develop positive habits

1. WebMD. What is metabolic syndrome? 2021. https://www.webmd.com/heart/metabolic-syndrome/metabolic-syndrome-what-is-it

2. Diabetes UK. Diabetes risk factors. 2023. https://www.diabetes.org.uk/diabetes-the-basics/types-of-diabetes/type-2/diabetes-risk-factors

3. NHS. Cardiovascular disease. 2022. https://www.nhs.uk/conditions/cardiovascular-disease/

4. Neal DT, et al. Habits – a repeat performance. *Current Directions in Psychological Science.* 2006;15(4):198–202.

5. Espeland D, et al. Health effects of voluntary exposure to cold water – a continuing subject of debate. *International Journal of Circumpolar Health.* 2022;81(1):2111789.

6. Duhigg C. 2014. *The Power of Habit.* London: Random House.

7. Kotronia E, et al. Oral health and all-cause, cardiovascular disease, and respiratory mortality in older people in the UK and USA. *Scientific Reports.* 2021;11(1):16452.

8. American Academy of Neurology. Taking good care of your teeth may be good for your brain. 2023. https://www.sciencedaily.com/releases/2023/07/230705171101.htm

9. Ward AF, et al. Brain drain: The mere presence of one's own smartphone reduces available cognitive capacity. *Journal of the Association for Consumer Research.* 2017;2(2):140–154.

10. Salk. Satchidananda Panda, PhD. https://www.salk.edu/scientist/satchidananda-panda/

11. Gardner S. Study focuses on strategies for achieving goals. Dominican University. 2015. https://www.dominican.edu/sites/default/files/2020-02/gailmatthews-harvard-goals-researchsummary.pdf

12. Griffin K. Interview with G Alan Marlatt. Surfing the Urge. *Inquiring Mind.* 2010;26(2). https://inquiringmind.com/article/2602_w_marlatt-interview-with-g-alan-marlatt-surfing-the-urge/

Path 8 – Continue learning for life

1. Nikolov P & Hossain MdS. Do pension benefits accelerate cognitive decline in late adulthood? Evidence from rural China. *Journal of Economic Behavior & Organization*. 2023;205:594–617.
2. Conner TS, et al. Everyday creative activity as a path to flourishing. *The Journal of Positive Psychology*. 2018;13(2):181–189.
3. Csikszentmihalyi, M. 2002. *Flow*. Revised edition. London: Rider.
4. Zawadzki MJ. Real-time associations between engaging in leisure and daily health and wellbeing. *Annals of Behavioural Medicine.* 2015;49:605–615.

Acknowledgements

Oh goodness, where to begin? There are so many people to thank who have helped me in my journey through life and through my journey to get this book finished. My parents, my three brothers, extended family, school, and friends shaped my growing up and I am so lucky that I still see many friends from primary and secondary school. A big shout out to the GANG! Growing up I wanted to be a doctor, and despite being fairly academic, the discovery of a social life as a teenager meant that my studies took a back seat, and I knew I was never going to work hard enough to achieve that goal. My second choice of studying biology and becoming a teacher did materialise and I have always loved teaching. I think it is the bossiness in me coming out! I know my colleagues over the years will be nodding their heads here. Thanks for putting up with me.

After teaching for six years I moved to Scotland with my husband, Dave, and my young girls, and I soon fell in love with Scotland and the new friends I made. Once the girls were a bit older, I was delighted to secure a position in the NHS working in Health Promotion. This was the start of my experience of training adults rather than teaching school children, and I soon learnt that I loved that too. And they were much better behaved. Well, most of them! When I moved into a new role in organisational development, still with the NHS, this was what really started a new path, which has ultimately led to this book. I want to thank Diane West and Helen Hellewell for believing that I could do the job and for introducing me to *The 7 Habits of Highly Effective People* by Stephen R Covey. Later my boss Vicky Irons supported me to train to deliver the 7 Habits programme, which was a pivotal moment in my career. I loved running these workshops, and this was hugely influenced by having two amazing co-facilitators, Joleen McCool and Wendy Simpson. Their support helped me to grow in skills and confidence. Having great colleagues and leaders makes all the difference at work, and I was lucky to have so many. Ed Wallace, our lead GP, supported me at every step and particularly nurtured my interest in how lifestyle can improve health outcomes, and we have great discussions about health to this day. Lynn Barker was a great boss and I have continued to benefit from her support ever since. Thank you. I would not have been able to do anything without the best admin support anyone could have. Suzanne Ogle, you are a complete star. Nick Haldane and Alec Murray were fantastic clinical leads who helped me grow in both knowledge and skills. There are so many great people in the NHS, so thank you to everyone who made my work there a time of learning and fun.

After working with so many wonderful colleagues at the NHS for over 15 years, I decided it was time for a change and moved to a part-time job at the University of St Andrews and set up my own business. This was rather scary but with

Dave's backing I took the leap. Joining my local St Andrews Business Club was instrumental in helping me feel that I was not totally alone in my self-employment world. Meeting Caroline Rochford, who had, like me, been a former NHS employee but who was now a successful businesswoman, gave me some hope that I would eventually get there myself. There are so many wonderful people in the Business Club, so a big thanks to all of them who have supported and influenced me as my business has evolved. Many of them have become good friends. Thanks to Caroline Trotter for my lovely headshot that makes me look years younger, and JJ Stenhouse, Audrey and Neil McNair, Jakub Bodys and Wendy Maltman (The Malting House) for your support with getting this book launched!

Once I decided that part of my business was to develop my own training courses, I had the brilliant support of Claire Eaglesham. I had met Claire while I was training as a coach, and she became my co-facilitator in my first tentative steps at developing and running my own wellbeing course. I could not have done it without you, Claire! I know I would have had very few participants at my first course if it was not for the help of Chris Lusk, who has an encyclopaedic knowledge and experience of student wellbeing. Your book next, Chris! Next step was an online course, and that was only possible due to the help of Business Gateway, who run workshops for small businesses. A great workshop on producing videos was invaluable for helping me get online. My course needed a couple of sketches to be acted out, so I persuaded Diane Munday and Lynn Neville, former colleagues from the University of St Andrews, to be my actors. I think they missed their vocations – they were stars. Once lockdown hit and we sheltered in our houses, it was full steam ahead with developing the online course. Here, the kind people who share their expertise on YouTube were invaluable. Sorry I can't give you a name check! What would small business owners do without these resources? Turning the course into this book was helped by coaching from Rebecca Wilson, who asked me the tough questions and who kept me accountable. She was writing her own book, so she knew what I was going through. I am certain that without her this book would never have been finished. Top tip – get a coach!

I have so many other people to thank for their part in my story. Gillian McMichael for being a great coach teacher and for introducing me to Joseph Grech, another fantastic teacher and my coaching mentor. Rosa Fricker for admin support and great patience with my random requests. Gail Smith and Lynn Campbell for supporting me in my new business. Belinda McDonald for sharing her mother's wisdom.

Many people receive my newsletter each month and enter my book giveaway or drop me an email. I don't think those people know how much their messages mean to me. Special thanks to Gary Scott for all your feedback on my terrible jokes. It is what keeps small business owners going. I am 5ft 6in by the way. No, the jokes never get any better! ☺

A massive thank you to all my clients. I have learnt so much from you and have loved meeting wonderful new people. To everyone who has commissioned me to work with them, or their team, or booked me for a workshop or talk, your faith in me is very humbling.

Writing this book has been a great pleasure. My main problem is that I keep thinking of more and more things I want to add in, but there comes a time when you have to stop. Getting the book from Word document to paperback or ebook would not have been possible without a number of very important people. Gillian McGregor, Judith Walker and Claire Maindron, who read the book as each path was completed and gave me feedback to improve the book. It was not just feedback they were providing; they were filling me with the confidence to actually go to print. Such a precious gift. The eight lovely people who shared their stories after having completed the *Positive Paths to Wellbeing* course (all names have been changed). I was glad that the course helped you, but you have helped me so much in return. Natasha Alonzi for her help with the nutrition section. My daughter Emily Carr for being the patient expert behind the diagrams. My lovely LinkedIn connections and newsletter readers who commented on and gave ideas for the book cover. My advance copy readers Helen Melvin, Rita Dick and Dave who picked out all sorts of things I had missed. My proofreaders, Hilary Buchanan and Claire Dignall, who have ensured that my book is as perfect as possible. That really is a special skill. Any remaining errors will have been caused by me fiddling with the manuscript.

When you sit and reflect on all the people you have learnt from over the years, it is very humbling. So many people share their knowledge so freely, and knowledge truly grows when we share information that can help others. Thank you also to the people who help to keep my wellbeing on track. To the Pinkerton Posse for being such great friends and for providing endless support and fun. Heather Bones and Tracy Knox for getting me away from the desk for a coffee and a laugh. Angela Anderson, Carla Guidotti Heron and the other Jeffers for keeping me running. Karen Robson, Brenda Spowart and Valerie Dickson for putting up with my terrible golf and my inability to play more than nine holes. All my Anster Allsorts running buddies as without you I would probably be a couch potato! Laurie Bell for being such a wonderful yoga teacher. You are my wellbeing champions.

Finally, I would like to thank all my family and friends for their support over the years. For their encouragement and belief in me. In particular, Dave for being my sounding board and putting up with regular proofreading requests when he has just sat down to relax, and my daughters Sarah and Emily for giving me permission to write about their teenage years. My family and friends are the reason that I want to live a long, healthy life. As I said in the dedication, this book is in honour of everyone I have ever learnt from. Thank you all from the bottom of my heart.

'No one can go back and change the past, but **you can** start today on a positive path to a calmer, happier, healthier future.'

About the author

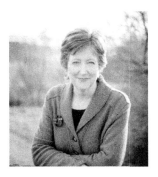

Marie Paterson is a wellbeing trainer and coach providing both online and in-person services. She worked in staff development in the National Health Service and university sector before starting her own wellbeing business in 2018.

Marie is passionate about supporting people to develop themselves and to live their calmest, happiest, healthiest life. She focuses on the whole person, to help her clients address different areas of their life as she firmly believes that all aspects of our lives intertwine and affect our wellbeing.

Marie delivers coaching, wellbeing talks, workshops, self-directed online courses and team programmes. She is trained in coaching, counselling, mediation, nutrition and exercise. Marie is an Associate Certified Coach (ACC).

She loves helping people make real lasting changes to their wellbeing. She comes from London and now lives in Fife, Scotland with her husband, David.

For more information visit www.mariepaterson.com

Printed in Great Britain
by Amazon

36534287R00138